OVER 125 NUTRITIOUS RECIPES
FOR A HEALTHY PREGNANCY

Natural
Pregnancy
Cookbook

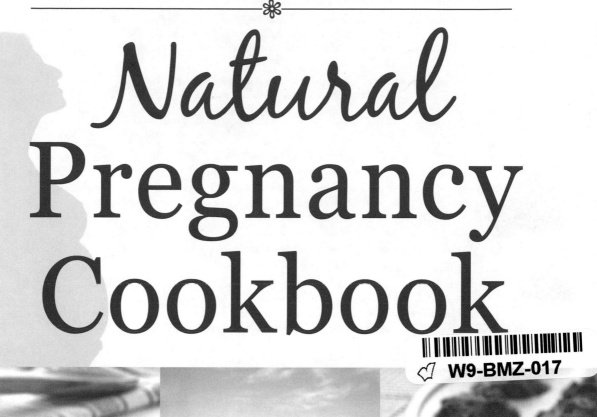

Dr. Sonali Ruder

Creator of the popular food blog *The Foodie Physician*

Hatherleigh Press is committed to preserving and protecting the natural resources of the earth. Environmentally responsible and sustainable practices are embraced within the company's mission statement.

Visit us at www.hatherleighpress.com and register online for free offers, discounts, special events, and more.

Library of Congress Cataloging-in-Publication Data is available upon request.
ISBN 978-1-57826-569-5

All Hatherleigh Press titles are available for bulk purchase, special promotions, and premiums. For information about reselling and special purchase opportunities, please call 1-800-528-2550 and ask for the Special Sales Manager.

Cover and Interior Design by Carolyn Kasper
Cover photo (center) by Adam Opris Photography

10 9 8 7 6 5 4 3 2 1
Printed in the United States

CONTENTS

Introduction   v

PART 1:
GUIDE TO HEALTHY NUTRITION AND PREGNANCY   1

    Chapter 1:   Pregnancy Nutrition—Eating for Two   3

    Chapter 2:   Planning Healthy Meals   24

    Chapter 3:   Morning Sickness, Cravings, and Other
                    Common Side Effects of Pregnancy   29

    Chapter 4:   Food Safety and What to Avoid in Pregnancy   37

    Chapter 5:   Tips for Eating Well during Pregnancy   49

    Chapter 6:   Healthy Cooking in Pregnancy   55

PART 2:
THE RECIPES   65

    Breakfast   69

    Appetizers, Snacks, and Sandwiches   97

    Beverages   133

    Soups, Salads, and Dressings   145

    Entrées   167

    Side Dishes   219

    Desserts   241

Appendix A: Know Your BMI   263

Appendix B: Dietary Reference Intakes for Pregnancy
            and Breastfeeding   265

Pregnancy Resources   266

References   267

Index   271

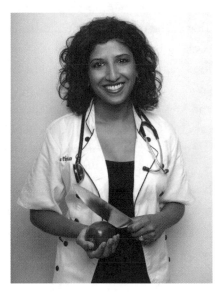

ONGRATULATIONS! IF YOU are reading this book then there's a good chance that you're pregnant. This is one of the most exciting times in your life and over the next nine months you will be filled with anticipation about meeting the little person that's growing inside of you. Pregnancy is truly a life-changing experience. Your body will be going through profound changes, and you need the proper nutrients to fuel those changes. You probably have lots of questions about what you should be eating to optimize your health and provide the best start for your baby. You may get a lot of advice from family and friends who want to share their own experiences. You'll likely hear conflicting information about what kinds of foods you should and shouldn't be eating and how much weight gain is normal. The truth is that recommendations about diet and nutrition during pregnancy are constantly changing as more research becomes available. This can be confusing and frustrating. Don't worry, you are not alone! Studies actually show that many pregnant women don't receive any advice from their healthcare providers on nutrition and proper weight gain in pregnancy. It's not surprising considering the fact that most doctors get minimal education on nutrition in medical school. In fact, the average medical student gets only about 20 hours of nutrition instruction.[1] This is really quite unfortunate considering how important diet is in preventing many medical conditions such as diabetes, high blood pressure, and heart disease. The good news is, by reading this book, you've already taken a step in the right direction.

I developed an interest in food and nutrition when I was doing my residency training in Emergency Medicine. After seeing patients day after day with diet-related medical conditions, I became inspired to learn more about the role a healthy diet could play in preventing those diseases. At the same time, I started experimenting a lot in the kitchen. Ten years after starting my medical training, I decided to further pursue my passion for cooking by enrolling in culinary school. That's where I learned the fundamentals of combining flavors and using different cooking techniques to create dishes that are nutritious and full of flavor. Healthy food can and *should* be delicious! Now my goal is to share both my medical and culinary knowledge with others, to empower them so that they can make smart diet and lifestyle choices. In pregnancy, this is even more important because what you eat not only affects your health but also the health of your baby.

Eating well during pregnancy means overcoming different challenges as your body goes through a myriad of changes over the nine months. In the first trimester, if you're in the majority of women, you will probably experience some degree of morning sickness. During these weeks, you may be less focused on a proper diet and more focused on keeping anything down. This is a critical time when many major developments are occurring in your baby. This book will give you practical tips on how to overcome your symptoms to ensure that you're getting the proper nutrition you need. Once the first trimester has passed, you'll enter what is often called the "honeymoon period" of pregnancy, the second trimester. After months of nausea, many women get their appetites back with a vengeance. All of those food aversions that drove you crazy may suddenly be replaced by intense food cravings. Hopefully you're one of those people who crave fresh fruits and vegetables but if you're not, then you may be prone to overeating. During this time, it's important to maintain a healthy diet while also not depriving yourself. We'll discuss what kinds of foods you should be eating and how much weight you should be gaining. Finally, in the third trimester when you're in the homestretch, your uterus is growing bigger and bigger and putting increasing pressure on your stomach and digestive tract. At this point, you'll probably have a difficult time eating large meals and will benefit from eating smaller meals that are nutritionally dense and satisfying.

This cookbook combines the science of nutrition with the art of cooking to give you the necessary tools to cook your way through a healthy and fulfilling pregnancy. It includes a wide variety of recipes intended to appeal to the novice or the seasoned chef. Not too confident in the kitchen? Many of the dishes in this book are easy to prepare and can be made in the same amount of time it would take to get food delivered to your door. One of the best ways to follow a nutritious pregnancy diet is to cook at home. When you make your own meals, you can control the ingredients as well as the cooking techniques. Cooking at home also creates lasting memories and brings families together. Getting into the habit now will set a good example for your baby and will instill healthy eating habits from an early age.

Drawing on my background as a physician, I've included information about the amazing physical changes your body goes through during pregnancy—some desirable and some not so desirable. This book also will provide you with the most important nutrition facts—the nuts and bolts about what you should be eating in pregnancy to nourish both you and your growing baby. As a chef, I wanted to be sure to provide a variety of delicious, nutritious recipes to suit a wide range of tastes. Your diet should be exciting and satisfying in pregnancy, so don't be afraid to try new recipes and explore new flavors. Studies show that what you eat in pregnancy actually influences your baby's tastes, so start developing your little foodie's palate now!

There's something for everyone in this book, including quick and easy meals, slow cooker dishes, freezer-friendly meals and plenty of vegetarian options. There are milder dishes for the days when you're feeling a little queasy, and full-flavored dishes for the days when you're loving food. As a mom, I know how busy life can be, especially in the months after the baby is born. So I've also included lots of practical tips about how to plan your meals and stock your kitchen. With the right tools and ingredients, you'll always be prepared to make a delicious, healthy meal even when you're pressed for time. Hopefully this book will be one you'll refer to for recipes long after your little bundle of joy arrives.

Following a healthy diet full of delicious, fulfilling and nutritious whole foods can provide many health benefits for both you and your baby. What you eat and how you treat your body during pregnancy can put your developing baby on the path to lifelong good health. And the good news is that it's not that hard! Just follow the basic guidelines set forth in this book and you can sit back, relax and enjoy this precious time in your life knowing that you are providing the best building blocks for your baby's growth and development.

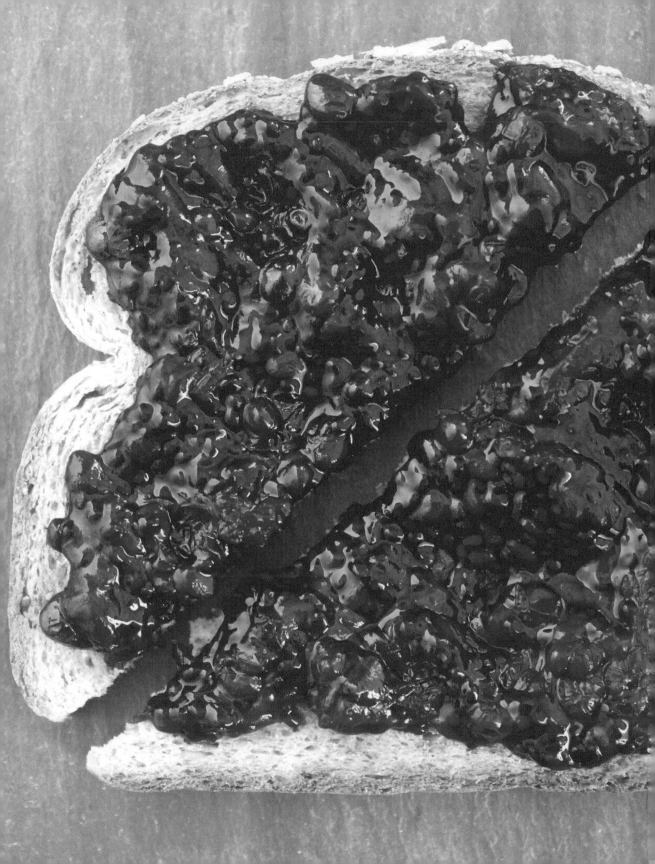

PART 1

GUIDE TO HEALTHY NUTRITION AND PREGNANCY

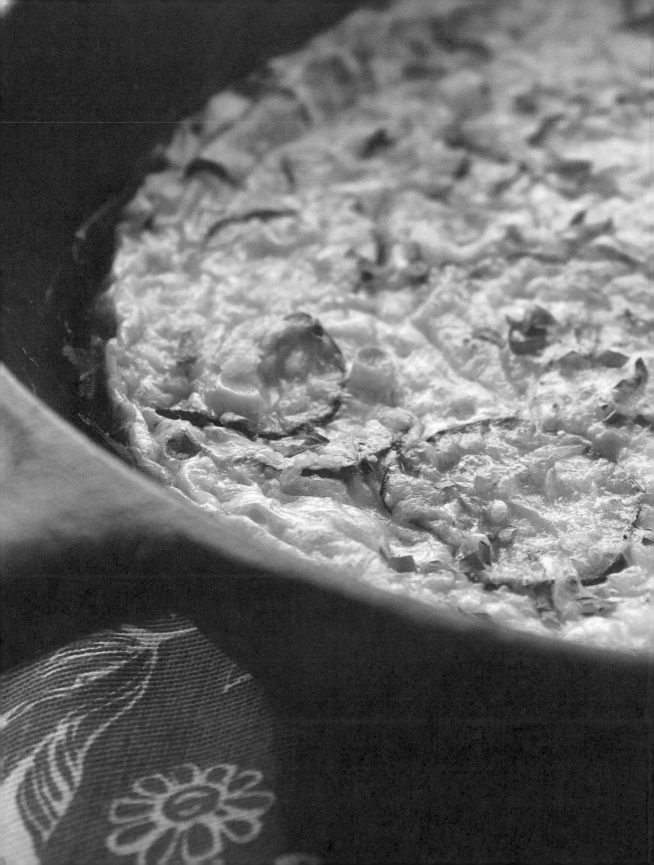

CHAPTER 1

Pregnancy Nutrition— Eating for Two

Following a well-balanced diet rich in nutritious, whole foods is an important aspect of a healthy pregnancy. It helps increase your chances of having a smooth pregnancy and also gives your developing baby the healthiest possible start in life. A healthy diet helps make a healthy baby. A growing body of research shows that your diet and lifestyle in pregnancy not only affects your baby's health at birth but can also affect their chances of developing conditions later in life such as obesity, diabetes, and heart disease. The good news is that prevention can start now as well.

If up until this point you haven't followed the perfect healthy diet or lifestyle, don't worry. For some women, pregnancy is planned, so they've had the opportunity to eat well, exercise regularly, and take nutritional supplements for months ahead of time. For others, pregnancy is a surprise. Either way, now is the ideal time to make some positive dietary changes, so that you can provide the strongest foundation for your baby's growth and development. The benefits of following a nutritious diet will last a lifetime (or two)!

Start by reevaluating your eating and lifestyle habits. This is the time to quit smoking, stop drinking alcohol, and limit your caffeine intake. Speak to your doctor about any medications you may be taking (including over-the-counter) and start taking a prenatal vitamin.

The best way to maintain good health throughout your pregnancy is to stay active and eat a healthy, sensible, well-balanced diet. Eating nutrient-dense, whole foods is more important now than ever! Now that you're pregnant, you need greater amounts of several nutrients like protein, folic acid, iron, and calcium than you did before pregnancy. You also need more calories.

You may have had people tell you that now you're eating for two. What that means is that you are in fact eating to keep your own body running while also fueling the growth of your developing baby. What it *doesn't* mean is that you should be eating twice as much. Think about it as *eating twice as smart, not twice as much*. In fact, if you are at a normal weight before pregnancy, then you only need about 300 additional calories per day during pregnancy.

What's more important than the numbers is what you choose to eat. Not all calories are created equal, so *eat smart*! Focus on choosing whole foods over processed and refined foods. Whole foods are foods that are as close to their natural state as possible. These nutritionally dense foods will provide important vitamins and minerals and keep you feeling full and satisfied. Try to avoid the empty calories found in processed foods like candy bars, potato chips, soda, and sweets. These foods have higher amounts of salt, fat, sugar, and other chemical additives to extend their shelf life and appeal to consumers' taste buds. They've also had many important nutrients stripped away in order to change their flavor and/or texture.

Did You Know?

A one-ounce bag of potato chips and a medium-sized baked potato have roughly the same number of calories. But the potato chips have about 65 times the amount of fat and almost 9 times the amount of salt as the baked potato. They also have significantly lower amounts of protein, fiber, and a host of other vitamins and minerals including Vitamin C, iron, and potassium.

Instead of buying snacks at the vending machine, choose meals and snacks that have a good mix of whole grains, dairy, fruits, vegetables, and lean proteins. To give you an idea of what an extra 300 calories per day means, here are some examples of healthy snacks or meals that are around 300 calories:

- ❁ 1 cup of oatmeal with ½ cup fresh berries and 2 tablespoons almonds
- ❁ 2 scrambled eggs, a slice of whole wheat toast and a small glass of orange juice
- ❁ 6 ounces nonfat yogurt with a banana and 3 tablespoons granola
- ❁ Baked potato with ½ cup broccoli, 2 ounces low-fat cheese and ¼ cup salsa
- ❁ 4 ounces wild Alaskan salmon with 1 cup broccoli and ½ cup brown rice
- ❁ Apple with 1 tablespoon almond butter and 6 whole grain crackers
- ❁ Small whole wheat bagel with 2 tablespoons reduced-fat cream cheese and 1 cup melon
- ❁ Turkey sandwich on whole wheat bread with lettuce, tomato, a slice of reduced-fat cheese and mustard

HOW MUCH WEIGHT SHOULD I GAIN?

So how much weight should you gain during your pregnancy? The recommended amount can range anywhere from 11 to 40 pounds (recommendations are different for twins). If that seems like a very wide range, you're right, it is! The current guidelines for weight gain during pregnancy, as recommended by the Institute of Medicine[1] are:

PRE-PREGNANCY WEIGHT	TOTAL WEIGHT GAIN RANGE (LBS)
Underweight (BMI <18.5)	28–40
Normal weight (BMI 18.5–24.9)	25–35
Overweight (BMI 25.0–29.9)	15–25
Obese (≥30)	11–20

So for example, if you were at a normal weight before you were pregnant, then it is recommended that you gain between 25 and 35 pounds during your pregnancy. If you were underweight before you got pregnant, your range is a little higher and if you were overweight, your range is a little bit lower. If you're expecting twins, you should aim to gain 37 to 54 pounds if you are a normal BMI, 31 to 50 pounds if you are overweight and 25 to 42 pounds if you are obese.

Just as important as how much weight you gain is the rate at which you gain it. You want to gain weight gradually during your pregnancy with most of the weight gained in the last trimester. Many women don't gain any weight in the first trimester because of morning sickness. In general, it's recommended that you gain about *2 to 4 pounds total* in the first trimester. Most of your weight gain will be in the second and third trimesters when you should gain *2 to 4 pounds per month* depending on your pre-pregnancy weight.

These guidelines were updated from the previous guidelines, which were almost two decades old. There were two major changes with these updated guidelines. First, the current recommendations are now based on the World Health Organization's (WHO) BMI categories. BMI, which stands for body mass index, is a measure of body fat based on your weight and height.

How to Calculate Your BMI

MEASUREMENT UNITS	BMI FORMULA
Kilograms and meters (or centimeters)	weight (kg) / [height (m)]^2
Pounds and inches	weight (lb) / [height (in)]^2 x 703

If math isn't your thing, you can look up your BMI on the table in Appendix A.

The second major change that was made to the guidelines was the addition of a specific and relatively narrow range of recommended weight gain for obese women. This is because over the past couple of decades, there has been a significant shift in the population of women having babies. American moms are more ethnically diverse nowadays, they are having more twin and triplet pregnancies, and they tend to be older when they conceive. Additionally, women today are, on average, heavier than they've ever been before. A larger percentage of women, nearly 60 percent, are starting their pregnancies overweight or obese and are gaining too much weight during pregnancy. This can lead to medical complications like high blood pressure and diabetes and can put both the mother's and baby's health at risk. There is evidence to show that excessive weight gain in pregnancy can lead to bigger babies, which also means a higher rate of Cesarean section.[2] It can also cause mom to have a harder time losing weight after the baby is born. Women who gain more than the recommended amount of weight and fail to lose this weight within 6 months of giving birth are at much higher risk of being obese 10 years later. Studies show it may also increase your child's odds of being overweight in the future.[3,4]

Obesity in pregnancy is also associated with a wide range of both maternal and neonatal complications such as an increased rate of miscarriage, fetal defects and mortality, gestational hypertension, preeclampsia, gestational diabetes and blood clots.[5]

Conversely, not gaining enough weight can put women at risk for complications like preterm delivery and low birth weight babies, which can also be associated with many medical issues. Remember, the guidelines for weight gain are in place to try to optimize the health of both you and your baby.

While it is important to know all of this information in general, don't drive yourself crazy with the scale! Your doctor will be closely monitoring your weight at every office visit and should let you know if you are gaining weight too quickly or not gaining enough. If either case applies to you, you may need to reevaluate your dietary intake.

Where Does the Weight Go?[6]

Wait a minute! Where does all that extra pregnancy weight go? Here's a breakdown:

* Baby: 6–8 pounds
* Placenta: 1½ pounds
* Amniotic fluid: 2 pounds
* Uterus growth: 2 pounds
* Breast growth: 2 pounds
* Your blood and body fluids: 8 pounds
* Your body's protein and fat: 7 pounds

HOW MUCH SHOULD I EAT?

When you're pregnant, you should consume between 1,800 and 3,000 calories per day depending on your pre-pregnancy height and weight. On average, a pregnant woman needs a total of 85,000 additional calories over the 40 weeks of pregnancy.[7] During the first trimester, your baby is growing rapidly, but she is so small at this point that you don't need any additional calories. Your energy needs increase significantly in the second trimester as your blood volume increases and your baby continues to grow. During the second and third trimesters, it's recommended that you have an additional 340 and 452 calories per day, respectively.[8] To simplify things, on average, you need about an extra *300 extra calories a day* over the course of your pregnancy.

Dietary reference intakes (DRIs) are recommended amounts of certain nutrients, vitamins, and minerals that an individual should consume daily. They are established by the Food and Nutrition Board of the National Academy of Sciences and are intended to be used as a guide for good nutrition. Don't worry about eating the dietary reference intake for each nutrient every day. Your body stores nutrients for later use. During pregnancy, the requirement for certain nutrients increases because a mother's diet must provide all of her nutrients as well as those needed for her baby's growth and development. Nutrients are substances needed for growth, metabolism, and other body functions. *Macronutrients* (which include carbohydrates, protein and fat) are so called because they are needed in large amounts. *Micronutrients* (which include vitamins and minerals) are so called because they're only needed in small quantities. This section will go over which foods you should be eating to fuel the changes that are occurring in your body and provide the proper nutrients to your baby.

Refer to Appendix B for a complete table of DRIs for pregnant and breast-feeding women.

MACRONUTRIENTS

Carbohydrates

During pregnancy, the recommended amount of carbohydrates increases by 45 grams/day to 175 grams/day. Carbohydrates are the body's main source of fuel. They are broken down into glucose, which easily crosses the placenta to the baby.

They can be used immediately to provide energy or they can be stored for later use. Many cells in our bodies (like brain cells) must have glucose to stay alive, which is why it's so important to get enough carbohydrates for you and your baby when you're pregnant. Pregnancy is not the time to go on a low carb diet. If you don't eat enough carbs, your body starts to break down vital proteins for energy.

Simple versus Complex Carbohydrates

Simple carbohydrates or sugars are small molecules of sugar that are easily processed by the body and provide a quick energy boost. They are found in foods like table sugar, high fructose corn syrup, cakes, cookies, candy, and sweetened beverages. Try to limit the amount of simple sugars in your diet as they provide calories with few nutrients. They also give you a quick high and then leave you feeling tired, irritable and looking for another fix soon after. Instead, choose complex carbohydrates like beans, whole grains, brown rice, fruits, and starchy vegetables like potatoes, sweet potatoes, and corn. They are a healthier option and contain important vitamins (especially B complex vitamins), iron, and fiber. It takes your body longer to process complex carbohydrates, so they are more satisfying and provide long-lasting energy.

Carbohydrates

* **Good choices:** Whole wheat bread, whole wheat pasta, brown rice, beans, lentils, fruits, vegetables, quinoa, oatmeal, multigrain cereal
* **Consume in limited amounts:** Granulated sugar, cakes, pastries, cookies, soda, candy

Whole Grains versus Refined Grains

Try to choose whole grains over refined grains as often as possible. The USDA Dietary guidelines recommend that at least half of the grains you eat should be whole grains. That's because whole grains have high amounts of fiber, vitamins, minerals, and antioxidants. So what exactly are whole grains? The official definition by the Whole Grains Council is: "Whole grains or foods made from them contain all the essential parts and naturally-occurring nutrients of the entire grain seed in their original proportions."[9]

Refined grains, on the other hand, are milled, a process that strips away the most nutritious parts of the grain. The refining process results in a product with a lighter texture and longer shelf life but significantly less fiber and nutrients.

Whole Grains

Amaranth, barley, buckwheat, corn (including cornmeal and popcorn), millet, oats (including oatmeal), quinoa, rice, rye, sorghum (also called milo), teff, triticale, wheat (including varieties such as spelt, emmer, farro, einkorn, Kamut, durum, and forms such as bulgur, cracked wheat, and wheatberries), wild rice

The typical American diet includes more than enough carbohydrates but most of it comes from refined sources. So most people are getting too much sugar and not enough fiber.

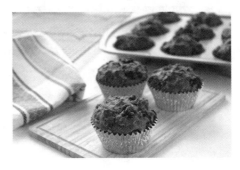

Here are some tips to increase the amount of whole grains in your diet:

❀ Choose whole grain bread or pasta instead of white bread or pasta
❀ Choose brown rice or wild rice instead of white rice
❀ Try substituting half the amount of flour in baked recipes with whole wheat or oat flour
❀ Use whole wheat bread crumbs or ground oats instead of traditional bread crumbs in meatballs and meatloaf
❀ Use oats or crushed whole grain cereal as breading for baked chicken, fish, or vegetables
❀ Snack on popcorn instead of potato chips or candy. Pop your own popcorn or buy microwave popcorn that has no trans fat.

Grain Definitions

* **Whole grain**—grains that have all of the parts of the grain seed (the bran, germ, and endosperm)
* **Refined grain**—grains that have been processed, stripping away some of the fiber and other important nutrients
* **Enriched grain**—refined grains that have had some of the original nutrients that were removed during the processing added back. White rice and white bread are examples.
* **Fortified grain**—enriched grain foods that have extra nutrients added. For example, many cereals and other grain products are fortified with folic acid.

Reading Whole Grain Food Labels

Labels can be confusing. To identify products made mostly from whole grains, look for the word "whole" before the name of the grain (example "whole wheat flour"). If this is the first ingredient listed on the label, then the product is most likely made from mostly whole grain. "Wheat flour" simply means it was made from wheat, not whole wheat.

Look for the Whole Grain Stamp— the Whole Grains Council created an official packaging symbol in 2005 to help consumers identify real whole grain products. The 100 percent stamp guarantees that the food contains a full serving or more of a whole grain in each serving and that all of the grain is whole grain. The basic Whole Grain Stamp means that a product contains at least half a serving of whole grain per serving. Note, while the labels are becoming more widely used, they are not on all products.

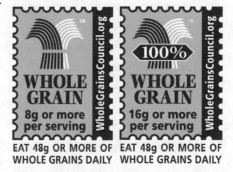

Fiber

Fiber is a type of carbohydrate that your body cannot digest. Fiber passes through your intestinal tract and helps flush out your digestive system. This reduces the incidence of constipation, bloating, and hemorrhoids, which are common side effects in pregnancy. The more fiber you eat, the more water you need to drink to keep everything running smoothly in your intestinal tract. Fiber also helps lower your cholesterol and helps decrease your risk of heart disease and

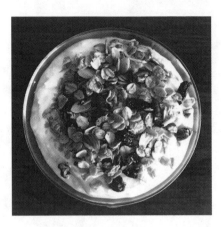

obesity. When you're pregnant, you should aim to get 28 grams of fiber daily, which is 3 grams more than the recommended amount for non-pregnant women.

Good Fiber-Rich Food Choices

*   **Fruits**—berries, dates, avocado, apples (with skin), pears (with skin), passion fruit, guava, oranges, bananas, and dried fruit (like figs, pears, peaches, prunes, raisins, and apricots)
*   **Vegetables**—artichokes, squash (like winter, butternut, and acorn), green peas, broccoli, sweet potato, collard greens, russet potatoes (with skin), parsnips, Brussels sprouts, beets, corn, spinach, and carrots
*   **Legumes, Nuts and Seeds**—split peas, lentils, soybeans, black beans, kidney beans, lima beans, navy beans, pinto beans, chickpeas, almonds, sunflower seeds, sesame seeds, pistachios, pecans, chia seeds, and flaxseed
*   **Cereal Grains and Pasta**— whole grain cereal, whole wheat macaroni or spaghetti, pearled barley, bran flakes, oatmeal, quinoa, brown rice, wild rice, whole wheat bread, rye bread, bulgur, cornmeal, and popcorn

Protein

Protein is the structural component of every part of both your body and your baby's body. Protein needs are greatly increased during pregnancy, with an additional 25 grams of protein daily above the recommended amount for non-pregnant women. This is because protein is vital for a wide variety of essential functions including the production of new blood cells, the development of your placenta, and the growth of your baby. This increase is also recommended in breastfeeding women because protein is needed for the production of breast milk. Most women, including vegetarians, will not have a hard time meeting the protein requirement because protein is found in a wide array of foods.

Most people tend to think of meat and dairy products when the word protein is mentioned but protein is also found in a number of vegetarian foods such as grains, nuts, and legumes (like beans and lentils). In fact, most animal proteins are high in saturated fat and should be consumed in moderation. So choose *lean proteins* the majority of the time like plant sources of protein, lean cuts of meat, skinless poultry and low-fat or fat-free dairy. Lean cuts of beef include flank steak, sirloin, chuck shoulder steak, brisket, tenderloin, and 93 percent lean hamburger. Although there are many cuts of pork that are high in saturated fat (like bacon, spareribs, or pork belly), there are lean choices as well such as pork tenderloin. To cut down on fat, trim meat before cooking and remove the skin from chicken.

Good Protein-Rich Food Choices

* **Meat**—lean beef and pork, skinless chicken, salmon, and other seafood, and eggs
* **Dairy**—milk (including soy milk), cheese, yogurt (especially Greek yogurt), and cottage cheese
* **Plant Sources**—tofu, edamame, quinoa, lentils, chickpeas, beans (black, kidney, navy, etc.), split peas, peanut butter, almonds, almond butter, pistachios, sunflower seeds, bulgur, wheat germ, and whole wheat bread

---

Greek Yogurt

The popularity of Greek yogurt has skyrocketed in recent years and for good reason. Did you know that compared to regular yogurt, Greek yogurt has about twice the amount of protein? That's because up to three times as much milk is needed to make Greek yogurt since it goes through an extensive straining process. It also has calcium and probiotics. It's a great pregnancy food, and a healthy protein-rich portable snack. Top it with fresh berries and nuts or granola. It has more fat than regular yogurt so choose reduced-fat or fat free versions. You can read all about the health benefits of Greek yogurt in my book *The Greek Yogurt Diet: The Fresh New Way to Lose Weight Naturally.*

Fat

Although so many of us are taught to avoid fat at all costs, your body needs fats to function. Fat is an essential nutrient to include in your diet when you're pregnant or breastfeeding. Not only do fats provide you with long-lasting energy, they are also necessary for your body to absorb fat-soluble vitamins (vitamins A, D, E, and K) and transport them to your baby. But not all fats are the same. During pregnancy, it's not about eating a low-fat diet. It's about eating the *right* fats. And some fats are crucial for the development of your baby.

There are four different types of fat found in food: monounsaturated, poly-unsaturated, saturated, and trans fats. Rather than trying to follow a low-fat diet, you should focus on getting the majority of fat in your diet from unsaturated fats, which are heart-healthy. *Monounsaturated fats* are found in foods like olive oil and avocados. *Polyunsaturated fats* are found in foods like vegetable oils, nuts, seeds, and cold-water fish. Try to limit the amount of saturated fats and trans fats in your diet as they can increase your risk of heart disease, high cholesterol, diabetes, obesity, and some cancers. *Saturated fats* come mainly from animal origins. Common sources are butter, cheese, milk, cream, meat, and poultry. That doesn't mean you should completely avoid these foods. Some of these foods (like meat and cheese) contain protein, vitamins, and minerals that are vital to a healthy mother and growing baby.

Just consume them in moderation. *Trans fats*, on the other hand, should be avoided. Most trans fats are the result of hydrogenation, a process that modifies unsaturated fats to make them more stable. This man-made fat is good for food manufacturers because it increases the shelf life of packaged foods but it's bad for your body. Trans fats are found in products like margarine, vegetable shortening, french fries, other fast foods, and many products on grocery shelves like cookies, cakes, crackers, granola bars, and many brands of microwave popcorn. Read the nutrition labels. If you see the term *partially hydrogenated* in the ingredients list, then that tells you it contains trans fat.

Sources of Unsaturated Fats

* **Monounsaturated Fat:** olives/olive oil, avocados, canola oil, peanut oil, sesame oil, peanut butter, and most nuts and seeds
* **Polyunsaturated Fat:** freshwater fish, flaxseed/flaxseed oil, safflower oil, grapeseed oil, corn oil, soybean oil, sunflower oil, walnut oil, and some nuts and seeds, such as walnuts and sunflower seeds

Omega-3 Fatty Acids

A specific group of polyunsaturated fats that are vital to the growth and development of your baby are the *omega-3 fatty acids*. You've probably heard a lot about this group of fats. There are 3 of them: docosahexaenoic acid (DHA), eicosapentaenoic acid (EPA), and alpha-linolenic acid (ALA). DHA specifically is essential to your child's brain and development not only during pregnancy and nursing, but also for the first few years of life. During your last trimester, your baby's brain goes through a huge growth spurt and requires very high levels of DHA. DHA is also crucial for the proper development of your baby's vision. In addition to being the critical building blocks for your baby's brain and eyes, omega-3 fatty acids have several other beneficial effects. They may help prevent preterm labor and may increase birth weight. They also help stabilize your moods and prevent postpartum depression. In addition, they may increase your baby's intelligence and decrease their chance of developing food allergies and eczema.[10-13]

Omega-3 fatty acids are not produced by our bodies so they must be consumed in your diet. The main food sources of DHA and EPA are fish and fish oil. Wild salmon is especially high in omega-3s. ALA is found in many plant sources like flaxseed and flaxseed oil, canola oil, olive oil, soybeans, tofu, walnuts, pumpkin seeds, dark green, leafy vegetables, and seaweed. These are all healthy foods with many important nutrients, so it's a good idea to incorporate these foods into your diet. But ALA hasn't been shown to be as powerful a health modulator as the two omega-3s found in fish. Our bodies convert ALA to DHA and EPA but the exact amount of conversion is unknown and varies from person to person depending on a number of factors. Many new products are available now that are ALA or DHA-enriched. Eggs are a common one. Omega-3s can also now be found in milk, orange juice, peanut butter, cereals, oils, pasta, and other products.

Scientific research is constantly expanding our knowledge of nutritional needs in pregnancy. Although we know how important omega-3s are in pregnancy, there is no specific DRI by the National Academies for DHA and EPA during pregnancy. As long as you get a good amount of DHA in your diet, your baby will get enough from your body during pregnancy and nursing, and infant formula and baby food are also supplemented with DHA. If you are at risk of not getting enough omega-3s in your diet, your doctor may prescribe a fish oil supplement with DHA/EPA omega-3s. This may be the case if you're a vegetarian, if you don't like fish, or if you live in an area with limited access to safe seafood (see chapter 4 for more information on seafood in pregnancy). Vegan omega-3 supplements made from microalgae are also available. If you do take a supplement, make sure it's from a reputable source and never self-prescribe.

Food Sources of Omega-3 Fatty Acids

* **DHA and EPA:** wild salmon, mackerel, anchovies, herring, tuna, sablefish (black cod), bass, trout, sardines, halibut, catfish, flounder, oysters, shrimp, lobster, clams, scallops, crab, fish oil, microalgae supplements, supplemented food: eggs, milk, soy milk, yogurt, bread, cereal, pasta, oatmeal, and peanut butter
* **ALA:** flaxseed/flaxseed oil, chia seeds, walnuts/walnut oil, canola oil, olive oil, soybeans, tofu, pumpkin seeds, dark green leafy vegetables (kale, spinach, Brussels sprouts, and watercress), and seaweed

MICRONUTRIENTS

Vitamins and Minerals

A wide array of vitamins and minerals are needed for the proper growth and development of your baby as well as for your own health during pregnancy. For many of these nutrients, the increased needs in pregnancy are easily met from the extra food you're eating. For other nutrients, the increased need is met because your body absorbs them better during pregnancy. But for some key nutrients, there is a risk that you may not consume adequate amounts without supplementation. Prenatal vitamins help ensure that you get all of the nutrients you need.

Folate

Folate is one of the most important vitamins needed in pregnancy. It's essential for the synthesis of DNA and for proper cell division. Low folate levels increase the risk of abnormalities in the formation of the neural tube, which forms the baby's brain and spinal cord. This critical part of the baby's development occurs very early in pregnancy (at about 3 to 4 weeks of pregnancy), often before a woman knows she's pregnant. That's why it's crucial for women of childbearing age to have an adequate intake of folate if there is a possibility she could become pregnant. The recommended intake for all women capable of becoming pregnant is 400 micrograms daily of folic acid. During pregnancy, that amount increases to *600 micrograms/day*.

Folate is important even after the neural tube forms. If you don't get enough, you can develop anemia. Inadequate maternal folate status has also been associated with low infant birth weight, preterm delivery, and fetal growth retardation.[14] Folate is found naturally in foods like dark green leafy vegetables and legumes. The American College of Obstetricians and Gynecologists recommends a prenatal vitamin supplement for most pregnant women to ensure that they obtain adequate amounts of folic acid and other nutrients.

Folic acid is a form of folate that is used in dietary supplements and fortified foods. In 1998, the U.S. Food and Drug Administration (FDA) and the Canadian government began requiring companies to add folic acid to enriched breads, cereals, flours, pasta, rice, and other grain products. This important public health initiative has greatly increased the amount of folic acid intake in our diets. Since the initiation of these programs, the incidence of neural tube defect has been reduced by almost 50 percent in the U.S. and Canada.[15,16]

Food Sources of Folate and Folic Acid

Spinach, asparagus, avocado, artichokes, Brussels sprouts, beets, broccoli, mustard greens, breakfast cereal, bread, rice, orange juice, pasta, wheat germ, quinoa, chickpeas, lentils, kidney beans, lima beans, soybeans, peanuts, liver, and yeast

Iron

Iron is necessary for making hemoglobin, the protein in your red blood cells that carries oxygen to your organs and tissues as well as to your baby. During pregnancy, your blood volume increases by a whopping 50 percent, so you will need much larger amounts of iron to make more hemoglobin. The extra iron is also needed to fuel the growth of your baby and your placenta. The recommended dose of iron increases from 18 milligrams/day to *27 milligrams/day* in pregnancy.

Many women actually start off their pregnancies with insufficient stores of iron, which can cause anemia. This is the most common nutritional deficiency in the world, during pregnancy. Iron-deficiency anemia can present with a myriad of symptoms including weakness, fatigue, dizziness, headaches, and shortness of breath. It can also have significant complications for the baby including preterm delivery, low birthweight, impaired cognitive function, and infant mortality.[17] For these reasons, iron is included in prenatal supplements. Also, just like folate, many grain products are fortified with iron.

There are actually 2 forms of iron: heme and non-heme. Plants and iron-fortified foods (like cereals, bread, and pasta) contain only the non-heme form. Meat, seafood, and poultry contain both the heme and non-heme forms.

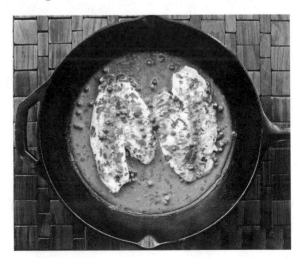

The heme form of iron is much easier for your body to absorb, so vegetarians have to be careful to get enough iron in their diets.

Food Sources of Iron

* **Meat sources:** beef, lamb, chicken, eggs, turkey, fish, shellfish, and pork
* **Vegetarian sources:** fortified breakfast cereals, blackstrap molasses, oats, quinoa, enriched rice, bread, pasta, beans (kidney, lima, navy, etc.), lentils, chickpeas, tofu, spinach, Swiss chard, baked potato with skin, green peas, kale, broccoli, prunes/prune juice, dried apricots, dried figs, raisins, and sesame seeds

---

Many compounds in foods can actually increase or inhibit the amount of iron you absorb from the food you eat. Here are some tips to increase your iron absorption:

* Eat Vitamin C-rich foods with your meals. Vitamin C greatly increases the amount of iron your body absorbs.
* Try cooking in a cast-iron pan. It will actually increase the amount of iron in your food because iron gets released from the pan during the cooking process. The longer the food is in contact with the skillet, the more iron it absorbs. One study found that pans released the most iron when cooking tomato sauce.[18]
* Blackstrap molasses is a good source of iron; try using it in baked goods instead of regular sugar. It also adds a rich flavor.
* Avoid drinking coffee and tea with meals. They contain compounds called phenols that interfere with iron absorption (see chapter 4 for more information on caffeine intake during pregnancy).
* Non-dairy forms of calcium (like those found in supplements or antacids) inhibit iron absorption, so take them in between meals. Of course, you should consult with your doctor before taking any supplements or medications.

Calcium

We have more calcium in our bodies than any other mineral. Ninety-nine percent of it is stored in our bones and teeth and helps to make them strong. The rest of our calcium is in the blood and tissues and performs several vital functions including maintaining a normal heartbeat, contracting muscles, transmitting nerve impulses, and clotting of blood. Given all of these important functions, you may be surprised to hear that the recommended daily amount of calcium does not increase during pregnancy. The recommended dose of calcium is *1,000 milligrams/day for women ages 19 to 50 and 1,300 milligrams/day for women ages 14 to 18*. This number does not increase for pregnant women because during pregnancy, our bodies become superefficient at absorbing calcium and absorb about double the amount.

Your baby has especially high calcium needs in the third trimester when baby's bones are growing rapidly and the teeth are forming. Unfortunately, most American women don't get nearly enough of this important nutrient. If you don't get enough calcium in your diet when you're pregnant, your body withdraws calcium from your own bones to supply your baby's needs. This decreases your bone mass and puts you at risk for osteoporosis. Low calcium intake also increases your risk of developing preeclampsia, a serious condition characterized by high blood pressure, swelling, headaches, and protein in the urine.[19]

If you're lactose-intolerant, vegan, or don't consume dairy products for other reasons, you can get your calcium from other food sources like calcium-rich vegetables and calcium-fortified foods. Calcium is added to many foods like orange juice, plant-based milks (like soy, almond, and rice milks), tofu, ready-to-eat cereals, and breads. If you're not getting enough calcium, your doctor may prescribe calcium supplements.

Food Sources of Calcium

Dairy milk, fortified soy, almond, and rice milk, yogurt, buttermilk, fortified orange juice, cheese (such as cheddar, mozzarella and Swiss) tofu (prepared with calcium sulfate), ricotta cheese, cottage cheese, ice cream, pudding, fortified cereals and breads, spinach, broccoli, collard greens, kale, mustard greens, bok choy, canned fish (sardines and salmon), almonds, almond butter, sunflower seeds, dried beans, tahini (sesame seed paste), and dried figs

Vitamin D

Vitamin D works with calcium to help build your baby's bones and teeth as well as strengthen your own. Calcium often gets most of the credit for building strong bones but without Vitamin D, it's almost useless. Your body needs an adequate amount of Vitamin D to absorb the calcium from food and supplements. The recommended amount of Vitamin D is the same for all women (pregnant or not), which is *600 IU/day*. Pregnant women

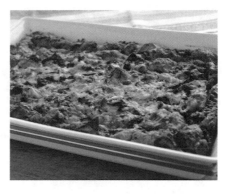

who are deficient in Vitamin D have a higher risk of pregnancy complications like preeclampsia. It can also lead to problems for your baby including rickets (which can lead to fractures and deformities), abnormal bone growth, and delayed physical development.

Vitamin D is one of the two vitamins (along with Vitamin K) that your body makes on its own. It's often referred to as the "sunshine vitamin" because our bodies make Vitamin D naturally from sun exposure to the skin. Theoretically, you could make all of the Vitamin D you need—just 10 to 15 minutes of sunlight exposure can provide 3,000 to 20,000 IU! But in reality, many women don't get adequate Vitamin D because the amount we get from sun exposure varies considerably depending on factors like geographic latitude and skin color.

There are relatively few natural food sources of Vitamin D. The best sources are fatty fish like salmon, tuna, sardines, and mackerel. In addition to natural food sources, many cereals, milk, dairy products, and juice are also fortified with Vitamin D. The U.S. government actually started fortifying milk with Vitamin D back in the 1930s because rickets was a major health problem at the time.

Food Sources of Vitamin D

Salmon; mackerel; halibut; catfish; tuna; sardines; tilapia; mushrooms; eggs; fortified milk; fortified soy, almond, and rice milk; fortified orange juice; and fortified cereals; and oatmeal

OTHER IMPORTANT NUTRIENTS

Although I've chosen to highlight some key vitamins and minerals, there are many others that play important roles in maintaining a healthy pregnancy.

Vitamin A is an important vitamin found in leafy green vegetables like kale. It's important for cell growth, aids in vision, and helps maintain a healthy immune system. It's also important for tissue repair in the postpartum period. However, excessive intake of Vitamin A can actually cause birth defects and liver toxicity. This is mainly a concern for women who take hefty amounts of Vitamin A in the form of supplements or eat large amounts of liver, which contains high amounts of preformed Vitamin A. For this reason, it's a good idea to minimize your consumption of liver during pregnancy. The good news is that the Vitamin A that you get from fruits and vegetables like sweet potatoes, carrots, cantaloupe, and broccoli is not toxic in large doses, so go ahead and enjoy these nutritious foods. They contain beta-carotene, which gets converted to Vitamin A on an as-needed basis.

The **B-complex vitamins** are a group of vitamins that help the body convert food into energy. They perform a wide variety of important roles in pregnancy that help support the growth of your baby. They are water-soluble vitamins, which means they are not stored in your body and must be consumed each day. Fortunately they are found in a wide variety of foods like whole grains, fish, eggs, meat, poultry, dairy products, leafy green vegetables, and legumes.

Vitamin C is a water-soluble vitamin that boosts your immune system, helps fight off infections, keeps your skin healthy and is essential for tissue repair and wound healing. It also helps boost your absorption of iron. Some foods that are high in Vitamin C are oranges, red bell peppers, broccoli, Brussels sprouts, grapefruit, strawberries, kiwi, cantaloupe, tomatoes, cabbage, and leafy greens.

Sodium and **potassium** are important electrolytes that are needed to maintain your body's water balance and blood pressure. They also play a key role in the contraction of your muscles and the transmission of nerve impulses. In pregnancy, your body needs more of these electrolytes to support the large increase in blood volume that occurs and maintain a normal blood pressure. But that doesn't mean you have to increase the amount of sodium in your diet. Most of us get much more sodium than the recommended minimum amount because it's found in high amounts in processed foods. Try to focus more on cooking at home with fresh ingredients like lean meats and vegetables and season your food to taste.

Iodine is a major component of the thyroid hormones and during pregnancy, your iodine requirements increase a good amount. Inadequate iodine intake during pregnancy can seriously endanger your baby's physical and mental development. Iodized table salt is one of the main contributors of iodine to the American diet but these days many people use specialty salts like kosher salt and different varieties of sea salt, which have a less harsh taste. It's okay to use these salts, but many of them are not iodized so be sure to also include iodized salt in your diet. Seafood and dairy products are also rich sources of iodine.

Choline is a nutrient that's essential for the normal development of your baby's brain. It's found in foods like eggs, liver, beef, pork, and wheat germ. Eggs are one of the most convenient sources but be sure to eat the yolk, which is where the choline and many other nutrients are.

Zinc is another mineral that's crucial for your baby's growth and development because it's involved in the synthesis of DNA. The recommended amount of zinc increases substantially in pregnancy. Good sources of zinc are wheat germ, fortified breakfast cereals, red meat, some shellfish, poultry, beans, nuts, seeds, whole grains, and dairy products. Like iron, plant-based sources of zinc are not absorbed as well as animal sources so vegetarians must be sure to increase their intake of zinc-rich foods.

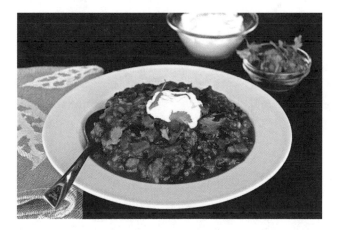

CHAPTER 2

Planning Healthy Meals

ALTHOUGH IT MAY SOUND intimidating, planning healthy, balanced meals is not difficult. MyPlate (www.choosemyplate.gov) is the current nutrition guide published by the United States Department of Agriculture (USDA) that helps show people how to make healthy food choices at every meal. While perusing the site, be sure to take advantage of their "SuperTracker" program, which gives you a personalized nutrition and physical activity plan. The program is based on five food groups and shows you the amounts you need to eat each day from each food group. Each individualized plan is calculated based on factors like your height, pre-pregnancy weight, due date, and activity level. The recommendations are given in measurements that are easy to understand like cups and ounces rather than the old method of describing amounts as number of servings.

MyPlate breaks down food into the following five food groups, which are the building blocks of a healthy diet:

- ✿ Vegetable group
- ✿ Fruit group
- ✿ Grains group
- ✿ Dairy group
- ✿ Protein group

Fats and oils are not considered a food group, but they do provide important nutrients. There is no minimum requirement for fats and oils. MyPlate also recommends a limit on the number of empty calories that you consume. Empty calories are the calories from food components, such as solid fats and added sugars, which provide little nutritional value.

To give you an idea of a sample plan, the following table shows a sample daily meal plan for a pregnant woman who is a normal weight (in this example, 5 feet 4 inches tall, weighing 125 pounds) and gets a moderate amount of exercise (30 to 60 minutes of moderate activity) each day.[1] It shows you how much of each food group you should be eating daily.

SAMPLE DAILY FOOD PLAN			
	1ST TRIMESTER	2ND & 3RD TRIMESTERS	WHAT COUNTS AS 1 CUP OR 1 OUNCE?
Total calories per day	2,000	2,400	
Empty calories	≤258	≤330	
Vegetables	2½ cups	3 cups	• 1 cup raw or cooked vegetables or 100% juice • 2 cups raw leafy vegetables count as 1 cup
Fruits	2 cups	2 cups	• 1 cup fruit or 100% juice • 1 large banana, 1 large orange, 1 small apple, or 8 strawberries count as 1 cup • ½ cup dried fruit counts as 1 cup
Grains (make one half whole grains)	6 ounces	8 ounces	• 1 ounce is 1 slice bread, ½ cup cooked pasta, rice, or cereal; 3 cups popped popcorn or 5 whole wheat crackers
Dairy	3 cups	3 cups	• 1 cup of milk, soymilk or yogurt • 2 slices hard cheese or ⅓ cup shredded cheese count as 1 cup
Protein	5½ ounces	6½ ounces	• 1 ounce lean meat, poultry or seafood • 1 egg • 1 tablespoon peanut butter • 12 almonds, 24 pistachios or 7 walnuts • ½ ounce seeds • ½ cup cooked beans
Fats and Oils	6 teaspoons	7 teaspoons	• 1 tsp vegetable oil • 1½ tsp mayonnaise • 2 tsp French dressing

SPECIAL DIETS

Vegetarian

Approximately 5 percent of the U.S. population follows a vegetarian diet, and that number keep growing.[2] With public campaigns like Meatless Mondays promoting cutting back on meat consumption, many people are eating more vegetarian meals even if they don't follow a completely vegetarian diet. You can have a healthy pregnancy if you're a vegetarian, you just need to make an effort to ensure that you're getting the right nutrients. The main concerns are getting enough protein, calcium, iron, zinc, and vitamin B_{12}. A prenatal vitamin will also help ensure that you get all of these important nutrients.

Fortunately, there are plenty of vegetarian sources of these nutrients (see chapter 1, for examples). One exception is Vitamin B_{12}, which is found only in animal products. Vitamin B_{12} is essential for the regeneration of active forms of folate and if you don't get enough, it can result in anemia. Some foods like breakfast cereals and meat substitutes are fortified with vitamin B_{12}. Women who eat even small amounts of animal products can easily meet their B_{12} requirements but most vegetarians (especially vegans) will need to take a dietary supplement.

Also, it's important for vegetarians to eat from a wide variety of protein sources. Proteins are made up of building blocks called amino acids. Animal sources of protein like beef, chicken, fish, and dairy products tend to be complete proteins, which means they contain all of the amino acids that are required by your body. Plant-based protein sources like beans, seeds, vegetables, grains, and nuts are usually incomplete proteins, which means that they lack one or more of the amino acids that your body can't produce. Eating a wide variety of protein sources ensures that you're getting all of the essential amino acids. There are some vegetarian foods like soy, quinoa, and chia seeds that are complete proteins, so keep these stocked in your kitchen.

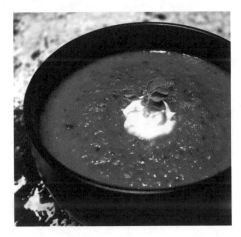

Types of Vegetarian Diets

* **Lacto-vegetarian** diets exclude meat, fish, poultry, and eggs but allow dairy products such as milk, cheese, yogurt, and butter
* **Lacto-ovo vegetarian** diets exclude meat, fish, and poultry but allow dairy products and eggs.
* **Ovo-vegetarian** diets exclude meat, poultry, seafood, and dairy products but allow eggs.
* **Vegan** diets exclude meat, poultry, fish, eggs, and dairy products

Lactose Intolerance

Milk is a great source of calcium and protein. But if you are lactose intolerant, you can get calcium and other nutrients from sources like fortified soy, almond, or rice milks. Many foods like vegetables, beans, and nuts also have calcium. You can also buy lactose-free milk. You might be able to tolerate cultured dairy products and yogurt because they contain less lactose and are often easier to digest.

Gestational Diabetes

Insulin is a hormone that regulates your blood sugar levels. When you eat carbohydrates, your pancreas secretes insulin, which signals your body's cells to absorb sugar from your bloodstream. When you have diabetes mellitus (DM), this process doesn't happen, so the sugar collects in your blood instead of being used for energy by your cells. Some women have preexisting DM when they become pregnant and others develop DM when they become pregnant, which is called gestational DM. According to a 2014 analysis by the Centers for Disease Control and Prevention, the prevalence of gestational diabetes in the U.S. is as high as 9.2 percent.[3]

Either way, it's important to work with your doctor to make a plan to keep your sugar under control. Gestational DM puts you at higher risk for having a large baby, which increases your chance of having a C-section and a longer recovery time after birth. It also increases your risk of developing preeclampsia. Your little one is also affected by this condition. It increases the risk of your baby having low blood sugar and difficulty breathing right after birth. And it also puts your baby at a higher risk of becoming overweight later in life.

Your doctor may recommend that you work with a dietician or diabetes educator to develop an individualized meal plan so that you know what kinds of foods you should be eating (and avoiding) to keep your sugar under control. It's important to monitor your blood sugar often as it may fluctuate significantly. Eat small, frequent meals to keep your blood sugar stable. Eat a combination of healthy fats, lean proteins, and complex carbohydrates with whole grains and high fiber at each meal. Staying active will also help keep your sugar under control, so if approved by your doctor, you should aim to get a moderate amount of exercise. If diet and exercise don't control your sugar, your doctor may start you on medication.

Postpartum Diet

The first few weeks after giving birth are usually an emotional and physical roller coaster. Many women experience a mixture of excitement, joy, and exhaustion. You will likely be sleep deprived and getting into the kitchen to cook a healthy meal will probably be the last thing on your mind. During this time, don't be afraid to accept help from family and friends with things like housework, shopping, and cooking. Get rest whenever you can. It's also a good idea to prepare ahead of time and stock your freezer with some nutritious, easy-to-heat meals (more on this in Chapter 6) so you don't have to turn to fast food.

You need up to an additional 500 calories per day as well as more daily protein when you're breastfeeding. You can do this by following the same basic eating guidelines that you did in pregnancy but just increase portion sizes. Don't skip meals and try to include a source of protein in all of your meals throughout the day. It's also extremely important to drink lots of water and eat plenty of water-rich fruits and veggies to make up for the fluid you lose during breastfeeding. It's crucial to get nutrients like calcium and vitamin D. Keeping up a healthy intake of omega-3s is also a good idea. It will help fuel your baby's brain development and may help decrease your risk for postpartum depression. Your doctor may advise you to continue your prenatal vitamin through this postpartum period.

CHAPTER 3

Morning Sickness, Cravings, and Other Common Side Effects of Pregnancy

BECAUSE OF YOUR INCREASING hormone levels, your body will be undergoing a lot of changes when you get pregnant. Although we are bombarded with photographs of celebrities in magazines flashing their baby bumps, the truth is that pregnancy is not always glamorous. You may experience symptoms like nausea, vomiting, fatigue, bloating, moodiness, tender breasts, and frequent urination. In fact, a lot of these changes may have started before you even knew you were pregnant!

From the moment when sperm and egg unite, your body goes into overdrive preparing for your baby's arrival. Your blood volume increases by about 50 percent in pregnancy, which means your heart has to work harder to pump blood to the rest of your body. At the same time, rising hormone levels cause your blood vessels to relax, which in turn leads to a drop in blood pressure during the first and second trimesters. Nearing the end of your third trimester, your blood pressure will return to its pre-pregnancy levels, if all is well. Your blood pressure will be checked by your healthcare provider at every visit to monitor for signs of gestational hypertension or preeclampsia, a serious condition characterized by high blood pressure, swelling, headaches, and protein in the urine.

Because you need more oxygen during pregnancy, your lungs will go through significant changes as well. The amount of air you inhale and exhale with each breath increases. As you get into the third trimester, your growing uterus will put pressure on your diaphragm and may cause some shortness of breath. Your stomach and intestines will also go through major changes, leading to some of the most undesirable side effects of pregnancy like bloating, gas, and constipation. Your joints will start to relax and widen as your pregnancy progresses, helping to prepare your body for childbirth. Even your skin, hair, and nails will undergo changes—some desirable (like stronger hair and nails) and some not so desirable (like acne and skin discoloration).

MORNING SICKNESS

Although it's referred to as morning sickness, nausea and vomiting in pregnancy can occur at any time of day or night. For some women it can last all day, while others won't experience these symptoms at all. Morning sickness typically starts early, usually around the 4th to 6th week of pregnancy. Between 75 percent and 85 percent of pregnant women experience morning sickness during the first trimester.[1] About half of these women will see resolution of their symptoms by around 14 weeks. For the rest, it takes more time to ease up. Some unfortunate moms-to-be will experience nausea throughout their entire pregnancies. It's impossible to predict how you will feel as every woman is different and every pregnancy is unique. In fact, the same woman can have completely different symptoms during each of her pregnancies. Although it's not exactly known what causes morning sickness, the increasing levels of hormones during pregnancy are thought to be a major factor.

The symptoms of morning sickness can be a lot more serious and debilitating than just a minor annoyance. For many women, it can seriously impact their quality of life. In a small percentage (around 1 percent), the symptoms can become so severe that they lead to dehydration and weight loss. This condition, known as *hyperemesis gravidarum*, requires hospitalization and administration of fluids, electrolytes, and nutritional supplementation through an IV.

Here are some tips for combating morning sickness:

- ❀ Avoid foods or smells that trigger your nausea. You may notice that you now have a sense of smell like a bloodhound. Perfumes, chemicals, foods, and smoke may all bother you. You're not just imagining it—a hyper-acute sense of smell is common in pregnancy. Unfortunately it can make nausea worse, so try to avoid those smells that make you queasy.

- ❀ Eat small frequent meals. In general, this is a good habit to start as it will give you lasting energy throughout the day and prevent fluctuations in blood sugar. It will also prevent an empty stomach, which can aggravate nausea.

- ❀ Keep snacks by the bed to eat in the morning when you first get up to avoid an empty stomach. Dry crackers and toast may help with queasiness.

- ❀ Hydrate. Drink lots and lots of water. Your body needs it.

- ❀ Give ginger a try. Ginger has been shown to help alleviate nausea. Some common products are ginger ale, ginger candy, and crystallized ginger.

- ❀ If you can't eat, try popsicles and smoothies. You may be able to tolerate them better than food.

- ❀ Stay cool. Heat and humidity may worsen symptoms.

- ❀ Consider acupressure wrist bands. These noninvasive bands are sold over the counter and apply pressure to acupuncture points on the wrist. Some studies show that they may help relieve nausea and vomiting in pregnancy.[2]

- ❀ A combination of Vitamin B_6 (pyridoxine) and the medication Doxylamine have been shown to reduce nausea in randomized trials.[3,4] There are also other medications to treat morning sickness like Metoclopromide and Ondansetron. Before starting any medications you should speak to your doctor to decide on the most appropriate treatment.

- ❀ Iron may worsen nausea. You can ask your doctor about taking your prenatal vitamin at bedtime with a snack instead of in the morning on an empty stomach.

Did You Know?

Doctors have traditionally recommended a diet of frequent meals high in carbohydrates like the BRAT (bananas, rice, applesauce, and toast) diet to help counteract the symptoms of morning sickness. But this advice is mostly based on historical anecdotal reports. In fact, some studies show that protein-heavy meals or snacks may reduce nausea.[5] Believe it or not, there are no randomized controlled trials that compare different types of diets to control nausea and vomiting in pregnancy.[6]

So what's the bottom line? You know your body better than anyone else so keep track of the foods you tolerate the best and focus on eating those foods. You may experience relief by cutting out foods with strong odors and spices, coffee, high fat foods, acidic foods, or very sweet foods. Try substituting snacks or meals that are bland, salty, dry, have lean protein, and are low in fat (like toast, crackers, pretzels, and cereal).

Fluids, Fluids, Fluids

You know that drinking fluids is important but what if the thought of drinking *anything* makes you feel sick to your stomach? In general, fluids are better tolerated if they're cold, clear, and carbonated. You may find it easier to drink in small sips from a straw. Sports drinks that provide fluids and electrolytes are also a good option. Some women find relief with certain aromatics like citrus and mint.

Here are a few beverage ideas:

* Cold gingerale (if it's made from real ginger, it will have the added benefit of reducing nausea)
* Ice water with a squeeze of fresh lemon or lime
* Iced tea with fresh mint leaves
* Cold sparkling water mixed with your favorite juice
* Homemade lemonade (see *Hydrating Honeydew Lemonade* on page 138)
* Smoothies (see *Mariya's Green Smoothie* on page 136)
* Popsicles—they're not just for kids! Try *Lemon Raspberry Buttermilk Popsicles* on page 258

PREGNANCY CRAVINGS

In the 2nd trimester, many of the aversions turn to cravings. These cravings can be intense, driving you (or your loved one) to make a late-night run to the store. Pregnancy cravings can run the gamut from pickles, potato chips, red meat, and spicy foods to sweet treats like ice cream, fruit, and of course, chocolate. It's not really known for sure what causes these 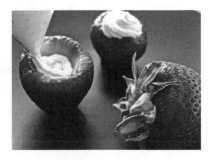 intense cravings. It may be hormonal or physiologic changes during pregnancy, but psychological and behavioral factors may also be involved. Occasionally, cravings can have potentially harmful health consequences. *Pica* is a condition where you crave substances that have little or no nutritional value like dirt, clay, laundry starch, and ashes. It's thought that there may be a connection between pica and poor nutrition, specifically iron deficiency anemia. If you are experiencing unusual cravings, contact your healthcare provider as they may want to test you for nutritional deficiencies.

Here are some tips to control your cravings without depriving yourself:

- ❀ Eat a good breakfast. This will help keep you full and prevent unhealthy mid-morning snacking.

- ❀ Eat frequent mini meals throughout the day. This will keep your blood sugar levels steady, helping to prevent cravings.

- ❀ Keep healthy snacks around so that you have something nutritious to reach for. Keep colorful, fresh fruit out on your counter where it's visible so that you're more likely to reach for it instead of the candy jar.

- ❀ Pack your lunch. While you're at it, pack a few healthy snacks, too. When you're busy at work and feeling fatigued, reach for your home-cooked goodies rather than hitting the vending machine.

- ❀ Stay active. Getting some exercise will help you feel good about yourself and give you more energy.

✿ Have an emotional support system. With all of the hormonal fluctuations occurring in your body, you may find yourself more prone to mood swings. Sometimes we eat to fill emotional needs, so don't be afraid to turn to family and friends if you need to.

✿ Get enough rest. When we're tired, we tend to reach for a sugary snack as a quick pick-me-up. It's important to get enough sleep before the little one arrives. It's not only good to help keep cravings at bay, it's also good for your developing baby.

✿ If your cravings are too powerful to resist, you don't have to deprive yourself. It's okay to indulge sometimes but when you do, enjoy it in moderation and practice portion control.

Healthy Swap Ideas

✳ Instead of potato chips, try air-popped popcorn or *Crispy Kale Chips* (page 119)

✳ Instead of a milk chocolate candy bar, try an ounce of good quality dark chocolate or *No-Bake Dark Chocolate Cherry Granola Bars* (page 110)

✳ Instead of french fries, try *Sweet Potato Fries* (page 226)

✳ Instead of a bag of cookies, try a handful of almonds mixed with dried fruit or *Tropical Popcorn Trail Mix* (page 120)

✳ Instead of ice cream, try an all-natural frozen fruit dessert like *One-Ingredient Banana Ice Cream* (page 256) or *Super-Fast Peach Frozen Yogurt* (page 255)

✳ Instead of Ranch dressing to dip your veggies, try *Simply Delicious Hummus* (page 114)

✳ Instead of a can of soda, make a healthy homemade drink by mixing sparkling water with fruit juice like *Pineapple Ginger Spritzer* (page 141)

CONSTIPATION, BLOATING AND GAS

These are some of the most common undesired symptoms of pregnancy, and the hormone progesterone is the main culprit. Your progesterone level is on the rise in pregnancy and one of its effects is to cause relaxation of the muscles in your intestinal tract, making them sluggish. As a result, food is digested much more slowly, leading to constipation, bloating, and gas. Once you're in your third trimester, your expanding uterus starts to put a lot of pressure on your intestines, further slowing down the passage of food and worsening symptoms. As if that wasn't enough, the iron in prenatal vitamins also commonly worsens constipation.

So what can you do about it? For starters, increase the fiber in your diet and make sure you drink lots of fluids. Increase the fiber gradually so that your body gets used to it—this will help prevent bloating and gas. Try whole-grain cereals and breads, legumes (such as peas and beans), fresh fruits and veggies (preferably with the skin left on) and dried fruits. See chapter 1 for more examples of fiber rich foods. Remember, fiber acts like a sponge and can worsen constipation if you don't accompany it with enough fluid so drink plenty of liquid to keep everything running smoothly. Get in the habit of carrying a water bottle with you. Prune juice has a mild laxative effect that can help relieve constipation. Drinking hot water with lemon is another natural option that helps stimulate your bowels.

Another way to help keep your intestinal tract moving is to exercise regularly (unless you've been told otherwise by your healthcare provider). You may benefit from a light walk after meals to help aid digestion. Avoid tight fitting clothing as it will put more pressure on your abdomen. Talk to your doctor before taking any laxatives or other medication. Reducing constipation also means reducing the chance of hemorrhoids, which commonly occur in pregnancy.

Because food moves through your intestinal tract slowly, you'll probably experience early satiety, which can lead to bloating, abdominal discomfort and gas. Eating small meals will help with this. Try to limit the foods that cause gas. For many people, foods like beans, cruciferous vegetables (like Brussels sprouts, broccoli, and cabbage), onions and garlic can cause a lot of gas. Unfortunately, these foods are all really good for you too. One tip is to rinse canned beans in a colander before eating, which washes away a lot of the sugars that cause gas. Cook your vegetables instead of eating them raw, as this may also help lessen symptoms. Try cooking with shallots instead of regular onions as they are milder than onions and may be better tolerated. (I use them in a lot of my recipes because they have a delicate flavor, cook quickly and work beautifully in sauces.) There are also over-the-counter enzyme-based dietary supplements that can help prevent gas (like Beano®). These are generally considered safe, but discuss this with your doctor before starting any medication.

GERD (HEARTBURN)

Once again, your pregnancy hormones are to blame here. Progesterone causes relaxation of the muscles that prevent the backflow of stomach contents into your esophagus. This can cause the acid in your stomach to shoot back up into your esophagus, causing a burning sensation referred to as heartburn. In the medical world, this is known as GERD (gastroesophageal reflux disease). Like constipation, heartburn often worsens in the third trimester because the growing uterus also starts to place a lot of pressure on the stomach, exacerbating the problem. To help combat these uncomfortable symptoms, eat small meals throughout the day rather than a few large meals. Take your time and eat slowly. Avoid heavy, greasy, or spicy foods as well as foods with high acidity (such as tomatoes and orange juice). Don't lie down right after eating as this will make the reflux worse. Try sleeping with your head on a couple of pillows at night to help lessen the reflux. Talk to your doctor before taking any medications. The good news is that the symptoms usually go away soon after the baby is born.

CHAPTER 4

Food Safety and What to Avoid in Pregnancy

THE FOOD YOU EAT in pregnancy affects not only your health but also the health of your baby. Just as it is important to follow a well-balanced, nutritious diet, so you must also consider the safety of the food you eat. It's especially important to pay close attention to food hygiene and to avoid certain foods when you're pregnant. This will help minimize your risk of exposure to potentially harmful organisms and substances that can adversely affect your health as well as your developing baby's.

Food safety is important for everyone but now that you're pregnant, it's especially important for you to learn how to protect yourself and your baby from foodborne illness. Foodborne illness is caused by eating food that is contaminated with bacteria, viruses, or parasites. According to the CDC, roughly one in six Americans (48 million people) get sick and 128,000 are hospitalized due to foodborne diseases each year.[1] That's a huge number! And pregnant women, along with their unborn babies, are at a higher risk for developing certain foodborne illnesses like Listeriosis and Toxoplasmosis. When you're pregnant, your immune system runs at low speed, which is a good thing because it prevents your body from fighting off your baby—a foreigner to your body—but it also makes you more susceptible to infections. Your unborn child is also more susceptible to these infections because she hasn't fully developed her immune system yet.

Some of the most common pathogens that cause foodborne illness are:

❀ *Campylobacter*   ❀ *Cryptosporidium*

❀ *E. coli*   ❀ *Toxoplasma*

❀ *Salmonella*   ❀ *Vibrio*

❀ *Listeria*   ❀ *Noroviruses*

❀ *Clostridium*

Most of these organisms cause flu-like symptoms like abdominal pain, cramping, nausea, vomiting, diarrhea, fever, headaches, and muscle pain. In people with a weakened immune system (including pregnant women), some of these illnesses can be life threatening. *Listeria monocytogenes* is a specific bacterium that can cause miscarriage and preterm delivery. Listeriosis can be transmitted to your baby even if you are not showing any signs of illness and can cause still-birth or serious health problems for your newborn. Unlike many other organisms, listeria can grow in refrigerated temperatures in products like refrigerated ready-to-eat meat products and unpasteurized milk products. According to the CDC, pregnant women are ten times more likely to get listeriosis than other healthy adults. If you suspect that you may have a foodborne illness, consult your healthcare provider.

The best way to avoid these pathogens is to practice smart food shopping, avoid certain foods that may put you at risk, and follow good food safety practices. As a pregnant woman, it's especially important for you and anyone preparing food for you to be careful with food handling and preparation. The best way to do this is to follow the basic rules of *clean, separate, cook,* and *chill* from the Food Safe Families Campaign.[2]

FOUR BASIC STEPS TO FOOD SAFETY
(1) Clean: Wash Hands and Surfaces Often
Bacteria and other pathogens can live all over your kitchen in places like your cutting board, sink, countertops, and utensils, as well as on your hands. This bacteria can then be transferred to your food without you realizing it. To help prevent the

spread of harmful bacteria, wash your hands for at least 20 seconds with soap and running water before and after handling food. Wash your produce, including fruits and vegetables with skin and rinds that are not eaten. This is important because the bacteria living on the surface of the produce can get transferred to the rest of the fruit/vegetable when you cut into it or peel it. Wash cutting boards, utensils, dishes, and countertops with hot soapy water after the preparation of any raw poultry, meat, and seafood products and before preparing any other food items. Bacteria can get trapped in the hard-to-clean crevices of your cutting board, so this is a good time to replace any that may be excessively worn out. You can also periodically sanitize your countertops and cutting boards using a kitchen sanitizer. You can use a diluted bleach solution made with 1 tablespoon unscented, liquid chlorine bleach per 1 gallon of water. You can also run your plastic cutting boards in the dishwasher (check to make sure they are dishwasher-safe). If using cloth towels instead of paper towels to wipe down surfaces, be sure to wash them in the hot cycle of the washing machine. When cleaning up juices from meat, poultry, or seafood, it's best to use paper towels and throw them away as bacteria love to grow on sponges and damp dishtowels. Clean the lids on canned foods and beverages before opening.

(2) Separate: Don't Cross-Contaminate

Cross-contamination occurs when pathogens like bacteria and viruses are transferred from one food to another. This is especially dangerous with raw meat, poultry, seafood, and eggs. To avoid cross-contamination, separate these items from other food items in your shopping cart, grocery bags, and refrigerator. In the grocery store, place raw meat, poultry, or seafood in a plastic bag to prevent the juices from dripping on and contaminating other food in your cart. Keep these foods in sealed containers or sealable plastic bags in the coldest part of the refrigerator. Keep eggs in their original carton and store them in the main part of the fridge, not the door, which doesn't stay as cool. Use two separate cutting boards—one solely for raw meat and one for ready-to-serve foods like fruits, vegetables, breads and cooked meat. Never put ready-to-eat food on a plate that had raw meat, poultry, seafood, or eggs on it without washing it with hot soapy water first. Don't ever reuse marinades used on raw foods unless brought to a boil first (although it's safest to discard the marinade completely).

(3) Cook: Cook Food to a Safe Temperature

The bacteria that cause food poisoning multiply fastest between 40°F and 140°F, which is why this temperature range is referred to as the *danger zone*. Cooked food is only safe to eat when it's been cooked enough to kill any harmful bacteria.

The best way to make sure that your food is cooked to the proper temperature is to use a food thermometer. If you don't already have one, you should consider buying one. They can be purchased online or at most grocery stores or home stores. There is a wide range of products from very basic to advanced. You can get a good basic one for under $10 and it's a handy kitchen tool that you can use long after your pregnancy. Even experienced cooks can have a tough time knowing how well their food is cooked by just the color and firmness. A thermometer removes the guesswork by measuring the internal temperature of a food. When using it, place the thermometer in the thickest part of the food, being sure not to touch bone, fat, or gristle. The table below lists the recommended safe minimum internal temperatures for meat, poultry, seafood, and egg products. Note that beef, pork, veal, and lamb roasts and chops should be cooked to a minimum of 145°F (with a 3-minute rest time) but ground meat should be cooked to 160°F. This is because ground meat has a higher risk of contamination. Bacteria actually live on the surfaces of the meat, not inside. When meat is ground up, the contaminated meat surface is broken up and spread throughout the rest of the meat, making the interior of a raw hamburger very susceptible to harboring bacteria. Cooking to 160°F means that *E. Coli* and all of those other pesky pathogens will be killed.

Seafood should be cooked to 145°F. Shrimp, crab, and lobster should be cooked until they're opaque. Clams, mussels, and oysters should be cooked until their shells open. Discard any that don't open. Eggs should be cooked until the yolks and whites are firm. Avoid sunny side up eggs, poached eggs, and sauces that contain raw eggs like Hollandaise sauce or Caesar salad dressing unless the eggs are pasteurized (more on this later). Poultry should always be cooked to 165°F whether it's whole parts or ground.

Food Temperature Guide[3]

These are the USDA-FDA recommended safe minimum internal temperatures. Use a food thermometer to be most accurate.

Fish	145° F
Beef, pork, veal, lamb, steak, roasts, and chops	145° F with a 3-minute rest time
Ground beef, pork, veal, and lamb	160° F
Egg dishes	160° F
Turkey, chicken, and duck (including ground)	165° F

(4) Chill: Refrigerate Promptly

Just like cooking food at high temperatures helps kill harmful bacteria, so chilling food to proper temperatures is equally important in preventing foodborne illness. Remember the danger zone (40°F to 140°F). Your refrigerator should always be set at 40°F or below because cold temperatures slow the growth of harmful bacteria. Your freezer should be set at 0°F or below. You can use an appliance thermometer to check the temperatures if you have any doubt.

Refrigerate meat, poultry, seafood, and any other perishable items within 2 hours of buying them (refrigerate within 1 hour if the temperature outside is above 90°F). Food should also be refrigerated within 2 hours of cooking. You don't need to wait for it to cool before refrigerating or freezing. When thawing out food from the freezer, never thaw at room temperature, such as on the countertop. The best approach is to plan ahead and thaw it in the refrigerator on a plate to catch any juices. If you're pressed for time, you can thaw food in the microwave using the defrost setting. Or you can thaw the unopened meat, poultry, or fish in a large bowl filled with cold water (don't use warm or hot water as this can cause bacteria to grow). Change the water every 30 minutes to keep it cold.

If you follow these basic food safety guidelines, you will be well on your way to ensuring your safety and the safety of your baby. Get in the habit of reading food labels when you grocery shop and check the "sell by" dates to make sure your food is not expired. When purchasing foods like meat, poultry, seafood, and fresh produce, give items a quick visual examination and a smell test before purchasing. Seafood, for example, should not smell fishy if it's fresh; it should smell like the ocean. Live shellfish like mussels and clams should have closed shells. If they're open, discard them. Check your fridge periodically and throw away any food that is expired. When in doubt, throw it out!

FOODS TO AVOID OR LIMIT IN PREGNANCY

Most doctors give their patients a long list of foods to avoid in pregnancy. What's interesting is that recommendations differ from one culture to another and even from one doctor to another. After all, pregnant women in Japan eat sushi and in France, women indulge in soft cheeses like Camembert. In the U.S., both of these are usually on the list of foods to avoid. On the other hand, pregnant women in France are often warned against eating fresh salads because of the risk of bacterial contamination, but this is not so in the U.S. Interesting, right? Many of the recommendations against eating specific foods like raw fish and unpasteurized cheese are to reduce the risk of infection by organisms like *Listeria, E. coli*, and *salmonella*. It's important to understand that most commonly, the contamination of food happens because of improper food handling. Even if a product is pasteurized, it can still get contaminated if the food is mishandled or not cooked or cooled properly. That's why it's important to buy your food from reliable vendors that you trust. Do your own research, talk to your doctor, and then decide what the best food choices are for you.

High Mercury Seafood

Fish and shellfish are rich in omega-3 fatty acids, protein, vitamins, and minerals and are an important part of a healthy diet. As discussed in Chapter 1, omega-3 fatty acids are crucial for the development of your baby's brain and vision, and seafood is one of the best sources of this nutrient. However, certain types of fish can contain potentially harmful levels of mercury that can affect your baby's developing nervous system. The amount of contaminants depends on the type of fish and where it's caught. Older fish and larger fish that are higher up in the food chain tend to have higher levels of mercury because they eat the smaller fish and therefore their mercury levels build up. Industrial pollution can also produce mercury that contaminates water, and for this reason, every state issues advisories about the safe amount of locally caught fish that can be consumed. Alaskan seafood in particular is among the purest in the world. Alaska's marine habitats are nearly pollution-free, which produces fish with superior flavor and texture. Alaskan seafood is also an environmentally responsible choice as its fisheries are managed for sustainability.

Both the Food and Drug Administration and the Environmental Protection Agency recommend that women who are pregnant or nursing should avoid high mercury fish. That doesn't mean you should avoid *all* seafood. On the contrary, go ahead and enjoy it but follow these guidelines: [4]

- ❖ **Avoid swordfish, shark, king mackerel, and tilefish**
- ❖ **Enjoy 8–12 ounces of low mercury seafood per week.** That's about the amount in two average meals. Examples of low mercury seafood are salmon, shrimp, pollock, tilapia, catfish, and cod
- ❖ **Limit white (albacore) tuna to 6 ounces per week.** Canned light tuna is lower in mercury.

These guidelines were updated in 2014 and are in line with the 2010 USDA Dietary Guidelines. What's interesting is that the main thing that changed from the previous guidelines (set in 2004) is that now there is a *minimum* recommended amount of low mercury seafood to eat per week (8 ounces). The previous guidelines only had a maximum amount of 12 ounces per week. The change reflects the growing body of research that shows how crucial seafood and omega-3s are to fetal growth and development. Unfortunately, an FDA analysis of data from pregnant women in the U.S. showed that we eat a lot less seafood than what's recommended. Of pregnant women surveyed, twenty-one percent said they ate no fish in the previous month. Of the women who ate fish in the previous month, the majority ate less than 4 ounces per week.

Raw, Undercooked or Contaminated Seafood

To avoid potentially harmful bacteria and viruses, avoid raw fish and shellfish like sushi and raw oysters. This also includes refrigerated uncooked fish like lox, smoked fish, or jerky. Cook fish to an internal temperature of 145°F as listed in the table on page 41. Pay attention to local fish advisories if you eat fish from local waters.

Raw or Undercooked Meat, Poultry, and Eggs

Cook meat, poultry, and eggs to the recommended temperatures listed in the table on page 41. In addition, avoid deli meats, refrigerated meat spreads, and pates or cook them before eating. *Listeria* loves to grow in moist environments like these. Avoid foods and sauces that may contain raw eggs like raw cookie dough and cake batter, eggnog, Caesar salad dressing, and aioli unless they're pasteurized.

Unpasteurized Foods

Pasteurization is a process that kills bacteria through heating. Some cheeses, especially soft cheeses like Brie, feta, Camembert, Roquefort and Mexican cheeses like queso blanco and queso fresco are more likely to contain unpasteurized milk and should be avoided. Firm cheeses like cheddar and Swiss are generally safe. For those of us that love cheese, the good news is that many cheeses are now made with pasteurized milk, so you don't have to give it all up. The take-home lesson is to make sure you read the labels at the grocery store and make sure the ingredients list "pasteurized milk." Milk, juice, eggs, and cider can also be unpasteurized so again, read the labels.

What is Pasteurization?

Pasteurization is the process of heating milk to a high enough temperature for a specific amount of time to kill pathogens that can cause illness. It was developed by Louis Pasteur in the nineteenth century. Routine pasteurization of milk started in the U.S. in the 1920s when people commonly died from infections that were transmitted through raw milk such as tuberculosis, typhoid fever, scarlet fever, and diphtheria. It has led to dramatic reductions in the number of people getting sick from these diseases. Pasteurization also slows spoilage and extends the shelf life of milk products.

Unwashed Fruits and Vegetables

To eliminate harmful bacteria, wash your fruits and vegetables, including those with skin and rinds that are not eaten. Avoid eating raw sprouts including alfalfa, clover, mung bean, and radish sprouts.

Thoroughly washing and scrubbing your fruits and vegetables under running water will also help decrease some pesticide residues (not all of them can be removed by washing). Now that you're pregnant, you may be more concerned about the effects of pesticides on your health as well as your baby's health. This is a good time to consider buying organic. It's a habit you'll probably want to stick with when you're ready to start making baby food, as well. Many pesticides can have harmful effects on your health and your baby's health, especially during the last three months of your pregnancy and the first few years of his life when his brain is growing the fastest. Studies have linked pesticide exposure to preterm delivery, low birth weight, pediatric cancers and even long-term neurologic development, behavioral problems and low IQ.[5-9] This is an area with a lot of ongoing research and every day we're learning more and more about the potentially harmful long-term effects of pesticides. At the same time, the organic movement has been growing in leaps and bounds as consumers become more educated on these issues.

In order for a food to be labeled "organic," it has to certified by the USDA National Organic Program as being produced without any synthetic chemicals or fertilizers, genetic engineering, radiation, or sewage. Organic produce does tend to cost more than conventional produce, but as the organic movement continues to grow, the price gap gets narrower. If you're on a budget, a good place to start would be to buy organic for those items that matter the most and to buy conventional for the rest. Each year, the Environmental Working Group, a non-profit group, publishes a list of the foods with the most and least pesticide residues, which they call the "Dirty Dozen" and "The Clean Fifteen." By choosing organic for the most heavily contaminated items, you can significantly decrease your intake of pesticides. Take a look at their website (www.ewg.org) and make the decision that's best for you and your family.

Buying Organic:
The "Dirty Dozen" and the "Clean Fifteen"

"Dirty Dozen" 2014—Purchase Organic

Apples, strawberries, grapes, celery, peaches, spinach, sweet bell peppers, nectarines (imported), cucumbers, cherry tomatoes, snap peas (imported), potatoes, (also kale, collard greens, and hot peppers)

"The Clean Fifteen" 2014—Safe to Purchase Conventional

Avocados, sweet corn, pineapple, cabbage, sweet peas (frozen), onions, asparagus, mangoes, papayas, kiwi, eggplant, grapefruit, cantaloupe, cauliflower, and sweet potatoes

Caffeine

The topic of caffeine in pregnancy often sparks debate and women sometimes get mixed messages about whether or not they can have caffeine in pregnancy. This is because many of the studies on the effects of caffeine in pregnancy are limited by small sample sizes as well as by other factors and many of the studies show conflicting data. However, the American College of Obstetricians and Gynecologists recently reviewed all of the scientific evidence to date and their current recommendations state that moderate caffeine consumption, which is *less than 200 milligrams/day*, will not increase your risk of miscarriage or preterm birth. It still remains unclear whether high levels of caffeine increase the risk of miscarriage, so it's best to avoid higher amounts. They also found no clear evidence that caffeine increases the risk of fetal intrauterine growth restriction (IUGR) but more studies are needed.[10]

So what this all means is that you can go ahead and enjoy a cup of coffee but keep in mind that the caffeine content in drinks varies a lot. How much is 200 milligrams of caffeine? To give you an example, an average cup of coffee can have anywhere from about 95 to 200 mg caffeine. Caffeine can also be found in many other products besides coffee like tea, soda, energy drinks, chocolate, candy, gum, ice cream, and over-the-counter medications. If you're a big coffee drinker, you may want to try to wean yourself off gradually to avoid the symptoms of caffeine withdrawal like headaches, irritability, and difficulty concentrating. You can also try mixing regular coffee with decaf and slowly cutting back on the amount of caffeinated coffee until you're all the way down to drinking just decaf.

Caffeine Content of Selected Products

Coffee, brewed (8 oz):	95–200 mg
Coffee, decaffeinated (8 oz):	2–12 mg
Coffee, instant (8 oz):	27–173 mg
Espresso (1 oz):	47–175 mg
Latte (8 oz):	63–175 mg
Black tea (8 oz):	14–70 mg
Black tea, decaffeinated (8 oz):	0–12 mg
Green tea (8 oz):	24–45 mg
Coca-cola (12 oz):	23–35 mg
Red Bull (8.4 oz):	75–80 mg
Chocolate chips, semisweet (1 cup):	104 mg
Jolt gum (1 piece):	45 mg
Häagen-Dazs coffee ice cream (4 fl. Oz):	29 mg
Excedrin Extra Strength (1 tablet):	65 mg
Midol Complete (1 caplet):	60 mg

Alcohol

Views on drinking alcohol during pregnancy have changed a lot over the years. Many of us (myself included) may have been told by our mothers that they in fact indulged in some drinks when they were pregnant. In 1981, when the Surgeon General started warning pregnant women about the dangers of alcohol, drinking during pregnancy quickly became taboo. Then in 1988, Congress passed the Alcoholic Beverage Labeling Act that requires all alcoholic beverage labels to carry a warning about birth defects.

While recommendations in other countries vary, the current recommendation by the American College of Obstetricians and Gynecologists is to abstain from alcohol completely during pregnancy.[11] This is because research shows that excessive alcohol consumption can lead to *fetal alcohol spectrum disorders*, a group of conditions that cause physical and mental problems in children. The most severe type is *fetal alcohol syndrome*, which is the leading known preventable cause of mental retardation.[12] However, there is not much data out there on the effects of light or moderate alcohol consumption during pregnancy and no data that shows it causes any harm to the developing fetus. Because there is a lack of consensus on what is considered a "safe" amount of alcohol to drink, the most common message pregnant American women hear is to avoid it completely. Some doctors however, tell their patients that it's okay to have an occasional drink. In many European countries, it's common for pregnant women to drink and doctors advise their patients to limit their alcohol consumption rather than cutting it out completely. It's interesting how practices change over time. The French government has now started requiring American-style warning labels on alcohol bottles.

What about alcohol in cooking? While it's true that some of it burns off during the cooking process, the actual amount of alcohol that is retained in the food ranges from about 5 percent to 85 percent.[13] This number is dependent on the cooking method and cooking time. A dish that's simmered or baked for 15 minutes (like a pasta dish) retains about 40 percent alcohol while a dish that's simmered for 2½ hours (like beef stew) retains only about 5 percent.

If you had some drinks before you found out you were pregnant, don't panic. This is actually quite common. Plenty of women have done it before you and have gone on to have healthy children. Now relax and focus on the rest of your pregnancy.

CHAPTER 5

Tips for Eating Well during Pregnancy

E ATING HEALTHY DURING PREGNANCY is very similar to eating healthy when you're not pregnant, except for a few caveats to make sure that you're eating the safest and most nutritious food possible for both you and your little one. The best plan is one that fits your lifestyle, provides all of the nutritional requirements for your pregnancy and ensures an adequate amount of calories to achieve optimal weight gain. Here are a few important tips to keep in mind:

EAT TWICE AS SMART, NOT TWICE AS MUCH

Choose fresh, whole foods that are nutritionally dense and nourishing. Fill half your plate with colorful vegetables and fruits. Choose whole grains like whole wheat flour over refined products such as white flour. Choose lean proteins, low-fat dairy, and healthy unsaturated fats. Eat plenty of nuts and legumes. Enjoy fresh seafood (for more information on seafood during pregnancy, see chapter 4). Avoid empty calories, refined sugars, trans fats, highly processed foods, and unsafe foods (for other foods to avoid, see chapter 4).

Pregnancy Super Foods

These pregnancy all-stars are packed with important nutrients to nourish you and your growing baby:

* Salmon (preferably wild Alaskan)
* Lentils and beans like black beans, kidney beans, chickpeas, and soybeans
* Greek yogurt
* Eggs
* Berries
* Sweet potatoes
* Spinach and other leafy greens
* Broccoli, Brussels sprouts, and other cruciferous vegetables
* Orange juice and citrus fruit
* Avocados
* Olive oil
* Quinoa
* Oatmeal
* Nuts like almonds and walnuts
* Flaxseed and chia seeds
* Dark chocolate

It's okay to give in to the occasional craving. If you try to follow these basic rules the majority of the time, you'll be in good shape. But eating a diet consistently high in high-fat, calorie laden foods can lead to unnecessary weight gain and may even program your child to prefer unhealthier foods. A 2007 study in the *British Journal of Nutrition* suggests that women who regularly eat a lot of junk food during pregnancy may be at increased risk for having children who become overweight because they prefer the taste of foods rich in sugar, fat, and calories.[1]

EAT SMALL, FREQUENT MEALS THROUGHOUT THE DAY

Don't skip meals. You should be eating about five times a day, starting with a good breakfast. This will keep your energy and blood sugar levels steady. Insulin is a hormone that regulates your blood sugar. It's also a fat storage hormone. If it gets too high (like when you chow down on sugary sweets), insulin signals your body to store those extra calories as fat. Constant high levels of insulin can also cause gestational diabetes. The more stable your blood sugar and insulin levels are, the more stable your weight gain will be throughout your pregnancy. It's also important to include a good amount of protein with your meals. Proteins take longer to digest than carbohydrates and thus help keep you feeling full for a long time as opposed to sugary snacks, which often provide a sugar rush and then an energy crash.

Why is it important to eat a nutritious breakfast? People who eat breakfast are more likely to eat a healthier diet overall.[2,3] Eating a good breakfast kick-starts your metabolism and keeps you feeling full for a long time so that you'll avoid overeating later in the day. It also increases your concentration and productivity throughout the morning. Eating breakfast also helps boost your intake of important nutrients like vitamins and minerals. Eating a bowl of folate-fortified cereal in the morning is one of the easiest ways to get in your recommended daily amount of folate when you're pregnant.

Here are some nutritious snacks and breakfast ideas that contain a good mix of complex carbohydrates, protein, fiber, and some healthy fat:

- ✿ Healthy Snacks:
  - ✿ Hummus and baby carrots
  - ✿ An apple or brown rice cake with natural peanut butter and a banana
  - ✿ 1 ounce of hard cheese like cheddar or Swiss with a handful of whole wheat crackers
  - ✿ 1 cup of Greek yogurt with berries or granola
  - ✿ A hard-boiled egg with a slice of whole wheat toast or pita

- ✿ Healthy Breakfasts:
  - ✿ Bowl of fortified whole grain cereal with berries and low-fat dairy, soy milk, or almond milk
  - ✿ Greek yogurt parfait with fresh fruit or jam and chopped nuts or granola (see *Sunshiny Day Breakfast Parfaits* on page 89)
  - ✿ Bowl of oatmeal with fresh or dried fruit and chopped nuts
  - ✿ Whole grain waffle or toast topped with almond butter and sliced strawberries or banana
  - ✿ Fresh fruit smoothie with Greek yogurt or tofu and flaxseed (see *Mango Peach Blast* on page 138)
  - ✿ Breakfast burrito, egg sandwich, or frittata (see *Summer Zucchini and Corn Frittata* on page 80)

Did You Know?

Many breakfast cereals are fortified with enough folic acid to provide 100 percent of your daily needs. Here are some examples:

GENERAL MILLS

General Mills Total® Raisin Bran
General Mills Total® Whole Grain
General Mills Wheat Chex™

KASHI

Kashi® Heart to Heart®

KELLOGG'S®

Kellogg's® All-Bran® Bran Buds®
Kellogg's® All-Bran® Original
Kellogg's® All-Bran® Complete®
   Wheat Flakes
Kellogg's® Low-Fat Granola
   with Raisins
Kellogg's® Low-Fat Granola
   without Raisins
Kellogg's® Mueslix
Kellogg's® Product 19®
Kellogg's® Smart Start®
Kellogg's® Special K®

MALT-O-MEAL

Malt-O-Meal® Frosted Mini Spooners
Malt-O-Meal® Crispy Rice

QUAKER OATS

Quaker® Oatmeal Squares
Quaker® Cap'n Crunch
Quaker® Corn Bran Crunch
Quaker® Cereal King Vitamin®
Quaker® Cinnamon Life
Quaker® Maple and
   Brown Sugar Life
Quaker® Quisp
Quaker® Toasted Oat Bran

HYDRATE, HYDRATE, HYDRATE

Up to 60 percent of our body weight is made up of water. All of our body's systems need water to function. When you're pregnant, you need larger amounts of water to support the expansion in blood volume that occurs. You also need it to maintain fetal circulation and amniotic fluid volume. Consuming sufficient water helps prevent many complications like preterm labor, dizziness, headaches, constipation, hemorrhoids, and UTIs. Watch out for dehydration! Keep an eye on your urine—it should be pale yellow or colorless. If you're getting dehydrated, it will become darker and more yellow.

The Institute of Medicine recommends pregnant women drink about 10 cups of water daily. How much you need depends on many factors like your activity level, your physical state, and the weather. If the thought of drinking that much water is daunting, don't worry. The recommendation includes all of the water in everything we consume, including food. Approximately 20 percent of the water we consume comes from the food we eat while the other 80 percent comes from drinking water and other beverages.[4] Think about how juicy a cucumber or piece of watermelon is when you bite into it. In fact, many fruits and vegetables are 90 percent or more water by weight. This is just one more reason why you should include a wide variety of fruits and veggies in your pregnancy diet.

Fruits & Vegetables with High Water Content

Fruits

Watermelon	Cantaloupe	Apricots
Berries (especially strawberries)	Peaches	Plums
	Pineapple	Apples
Grapefruit	Oranges	

Vegetables

Cucumber	Radishes	Spinach
Lettuce (especially iceberg)	Tomatoes	Broccoli
Celery	Bell peppers (especially green)	
Zucchini	Cauliflower	

STAY ACTIVE

Exercise improves your physical and mental well-being. Here are just some of the many benefits that exercise has for you and your baby:

- ✿ Lowers your risk of developing gestational diabetes
- ✿ Lessens joint and back pain
- ✿ Stabilizes your mood and helps prevent depression
- ✿ Prevents constipation
- ✿ Eases morning sickness
- ✿ Improves your quality of sleep
- ✿ Improves your balance
- ✿ Improves bone density
- ✿ Boosts your immune system
- ✿ Helps prepare your body for labor
- ✿ Optimizes your weight gain and lowers the chances of your child becoming obese
- ✿ Helps you get back into shape after delivery

According to the *Physical Activity Guidelines for Americans*, pregnant women should get about 2½ hours of moderate intensity aerobic physical activity per week during pregnancy and in the postpartum period.[5] Activities like walking, swimming, cycling on a stationary bike, yoga, and water aerobics are all good options. Avoid any sports with excessive bouncing, jarring, or stretching movements and any activity with a potential for falling. Remember, as your belly grows, it alters your center of gravity and your balance. As you get further into your pregnancy, avoid activities that have you lying flat on your back as it may decrease blood flow to your uterus. Make sure you stay cool and exercise in an area with air conditioning or good ventilation to avoid getting overheated. Once again, stay hydrated! If you were not physically active before pregnancy, gradually increase your level of activity over time. Know your limits and don't overdo it.

It's very important that you discuss with your healthcare provider how much physical activity you should be getting. In certain cases, your doctor may advise you to limit your activity. But in general, unless they have a medical condition for which their physician has advised them to avoid physical activity, most women can begin or continue moderate exercise during pregnancy.

CHAPTER 6

Healthy Cooking in Pregnancy

THE KEY TO EATING a healthy pregnancy diet can be broken down into three main principles:

- ❀ Cook at home
- ❀ Plan your meals
- ❀ Stock your kitchen well

COOK AT HOME

One of the best ways to eat a nutritious diet is to cook at home. There's no question that cooking at home is healthier than eating out. When you cook at home, you can choose the ingredients you use as well as your cooking techniques. Restaurant chefs and food producers use higher amounts of salt, fat, and sugar to make their food taste better to consumers. Cooking at home allows you to control these ingredients and make healthier choices. When you're in the kitchen, you can focus on using fresh, whole foods that retain all of the beneficial nutrients that are stripped away in processed foods. Over the last few decades, portion sizes in fast food restaurants have increased considerably. Preparing food at home also allows you to control how much you eat to prevent overeating.

Cooking doesn't have to be hard. You may find the thought of cooking dinner so daunting that you'd rather pick up a phone and order in. But the truth is that you can cook a healthy meal in the same amount of time it takes to get food delivered to your front door. Cooking at home also saves money. Packaged and prepared meals cost considerably more than cooking with raw ingredients at home. You can also increase your savings by packing up leftovers to take to work for lunch the next day instead of buying food out.

Use healthy cooking techniques. Try grilling, sautéing, poaching, and roasting your food instead of higher fat cooking methods like deep-frying. If you don't have the luxury of an outdoor grill, consider investing in a grill pan to use on your stove. It allows you to enjoy healthy, grilled dishes all year. Sautéing is a classic French cooking technique that involves cooking food in a pan at high heat in a small amount of oil. It has the benefit of being a quick cooking method and it allows the food you're cooking to get nicely browned while sealing in the moisture and flavor. Stir-frying is a similar healthy cooking technique that's common in Asian cooking and is perfect for quick weeknight meals. Poaching is a versatile cooking technique that involves simmering food in a liquid like water, stock, milk, or wine. It's commonly used with fish, eggs, fruit, and chicken and produces a very moist, evenly cooked product. It's a very healthy way to cook because it uses no fat. Roasting uses the hot, dry heat of the oven to cook food. It browns and caramelizes the surface of the food, which develops complex flavors and aromas.

Use olive oil for the majority of your cooking. However, if you're cooking at really high heat, olive oil may not be the best choice because it doesn't have a very high smoke point (the temperature at which an oil begins to burn). It also may not be the best choice when you're cooking delicately flavored dishes like cakes that require a more neutral-flavored oil. In these cases, choose oils that have a neutral flavor and higher smoke point like safflower, canola, peanut, or grapeseed oil. Canola is made specifically to produce a favorable fatty acid profile but keep in mind that the vast majority of canola oil is genetically engineered from the rapeseed plant. If GMOs (genetically modified organisms) are something you wish to avoid, choose a Non-GMO Project Verified product or substitute a different oil.

Besides all of the health and financial benefits of cooking at home, it's also a good habit to get into because cooking brings families together. For many of us, some of our most treasured early memories revolve around food, whether it be the festive holiday meals we shared with our families or the favorite dish our moms would whip up for us on special occasions. I hope this book will provide you with the recipes and tools to help you enjoy many family meals together so that you can create new traditions in your family. Cooking at home will help set a good example for your baby and start instilling healthy eating habits in him or her at an early age. Once he or she is old enough to join you in the kitchen, teaching your children to cook is a gift of health that they will use for their entire lives.

PLAN YOUR MEALS

The concept of meal planning is one of my biggest time, money, and stress saving tips. If you're not familiar with the concept, meal planning simply involves taking a little time at the beginning of the week to plan out your meals for the rest of the week. If you feel like you don't have the time to do this, trust me when I say that investing this small amount of time will save you *loads* of time later on. How many times have you stood there looking into your fridge, wondering what to make for dinner? How often do you make last-minute runs to the grocery store to pick up one or two ingredients for a recipe? How often do you end up throwing out ingredients that you buy for one recipe? Planning your meals will help you avoid these situations. It will also help you eat a wider variety of nutritious meals and cut down on waste, too.

Here's how it works. On the weekend, sit down and write out the meals you're going to make that week. You don't have to cook seven days a week. If you're a beginner, start with a more reasonable goal that works for you. Try a wide variety of meals and use seasonal ingredients to maximize flavor and save money. Try to make dishes that use similar ingredients to get the most bang for your buck. For example, if you're going to buy a container of miso paste to make *Quick and Easy Miso Glazed Salmon* (page 168), plan to also make *Miso Roasted Brussels Sprouts* (page 220) later in the week. Cook in large batches so that you have leftovers to enjoy for two or three days. Plan to eat those leftovers on the days when you know you're going to be the busiest. I like to follow the philosophy of "cook once, eat twice." This means making a dish like pulled chicken or turkey chili and transforming the leftovers into a completely different dish the next day. For example, the chicken in *Slow Cooker Pulled Chicken* (page 183) tastes great the next day sandwiched between two tortillas with cheddar cheese for a quick and easy quesadilla.

Once your menu for the week is set, make a grocery list. One of the tips I learned from interning in the test kitchen at a food magazine was to make an organized and efficient grocery list. It may sound unnecessary, but it will save you from wandering around the grocery store trying to find ingredients. Break the list down into sections (like produce, bakery, dairy, meat, frozen, pantry, etc.) and group your items into the sections. Cross them off as you shop. With meal planning, you should ideally be able to get everything you need for the week with only one trip to the grocery store. This will save you time and money and cut down on stress.

When you get home from the grocery store, follow a few tips to save you time later in the week and reduce waste. Wash your herbs, wrap them in a paper towel and store them in plastic bags to prolong shelf life. Follow the restaurant rule of FIFO (first in, first out) to reduce waste. When you're buying new groceries like milk or yogurt, put the newer food behind the older food so the older food is used first. Of course, always be sure to check the "use by" date to assure proper food safety and freshness. Buying family sized packages of meat like chicken will save you money, but if you're freezing it, break it down into single or double serving portions before placing them in the freezer. This way, you won't have to defrost a whole package of chicken to cook just two breasts.

STOCK YOUR KITCHEN WELL

Having a well-stocked kitchen is one of the keys to easy, nutritious, stress-free cooking. If you have the proper tools and ingredients, you can make delicious, healthy meals without having to run to the grocery store for last-minute ingredients. In addition to stocking your pantry and fridge, stock your freezer too. It's always a relief to open your freezer on busy days and find a home-cooked meal that just needs to be popped in the oven. Before I became a mom, I didn't really use my freezer much, but now I can't live without it! Your freezer will be your best friend once the baby arrives and you start storing breast milk, baby food, and so on. The first few months after the baby is born will be a whirlwind as you try to figure out how to nourish and care for this tiny little being. Now would be a great time to freeze some nutritious meals so that you can make sure you'll be taken care of, too. Be sure to make a habit of labeling and dating everything you freeze.

ESSENTIAL KITCHEN TOOLS

- ✿ Knives: chef's knife, paring knife, kitchen shears
- ✿ Pots and pans: large and small sauté pans, grill pan, large pasta pot (ideally with a steamer insert to steam vegetables), cast-iron skillet is also a plus
- ✿ Baking: sheet pans, hand mixer or stand mixer, spatula, a set of measuring cups and spoons, whisk
- ✿ Immersion blender or standing blender: for soups and smoothies
- ✿ Food processor or mini chopper (especially useful if you don't like chopping); consider an all-in-one tool with mini chopper and immersion blender
- ✿ Food thermometer: the best way to ensure your food is cooked to the proper temperature
- ✿ Tongs: the workhorse of the kitchen
- ✿ Heat resistant spoons
- ✿ Microplane zester/grater
- ✿ Two cutting boards: one for meat and one for everything else
- ✿ Colander: to rinse your fruits and vegetables, drain and rinse beans and to drain pasta (if you don't have a pot with a pasta insert)
- ✿ Olive oil sprayer (uses less oil to cut calories and fat)

ESSENTIAL FOODS

Pantry

- ✿ Cereal, grains and bread:
  - ✿ Fortified whole grain breakfast cereal (watch the sugar content); look for cereals that supply 100% of your recommended daily folic acid
  - ✿ Whole grain bread (look for the seal), whole grain wraps or tortillas, English muffins, or sandwich rounds
  - ✿ Breadcrumbs: whole wheat and panko
  - ✿ White whole wheat flour (it has all the benefits of whole grains but has a more delicate texture), enriched unbleached all-purpose flour
  - ✿ Rolled oats, quick-cooking oats, instant fortified oatmeal (low sugar)
  - ✿ Dried whole wheat pasta; multigrain pasta like Barilla Plus is another good choice if you don't like the taste or texture of whole wheat
  - ✿ Rice (brown and white): regular and instant
  - ✿ Quinoa

- ✿ Popcorn: buy popcorn and pop it in an air popper or on the stove-top; if buying microwave popcorn, make sure it has no trans fat
- ✿ Whole grain crackers, pretzels
- ✿ Wheat germ
- ✿ Oil, vinegar and spices:
  - ✿ Oil
    - Olive oil
    - Neutral-flavored oils like safflower, grapeseed, peanut, or canola
    - Sesame oil
    - Coconut oil: I use it mainly in baking recipes as a substitute for butter. It is high in saturated fat but contains compounds that may have health benefits
  - ✿ Vinegar: balsamic, cider, red, white, rice
  - ✿ Salt (iodized salt and kosher salt), pepper, and dried spices
- ✿ Nuts, seeds and legumes:
  - ✿ Whole, unsalted almonds, sliced or slivered almonds, walnuts, pecans, pine nuts, natural almond butter, and peanut butter (avoid brands with hydrogenated oil)
  - ✿ Flaxseed (and/or flaxseed oil)
  - ✿ Chia seeds
  - ✿ Sunflower seeds, sesame seeds
  - ✿ Beans: black, kidney, white, cannellini, navy, pinto, garbanzo (chickpeas)
  - ✿ Lentils
- ✿ Sweeteners
  - ✿ Sugar: unrefined sugars are preferred like coconut palm sugar or muscovado sugar; also granulated white sugar and brown sugar
  - ✿ Honey
  - ✿ Maple syrup
  - ✿ Molasses
- ✿ Baking:
  - ✿ Baking powder, baking soda
  - ✿ Vanilla extract
  - ✿ Good quality dark chocolate (preferably 70% cacao or higher)
  - ✿ Unsweetened cocoa powder
  - ✿ Unsweetened shredded coconut

- ❂ Other:
  - ❂ Low-sodium chicken and/or vegetable stock
  - ❂ Canned tomatoes: whole, crushed
  - ❂ Jarred salsa
  - ❂ Dried fruit: cranberries, cherries, apricots, prunes, dates, raisins
  - ❂ Crystallized ginger
  - ❂ Mediterranean staples: sundried tomatoes, artichoke hearts, capers, olives, roasted red peppers, anchovies or anchovy paste
  - ❂ Asian staples: low-sodium soy sauce or tamari (gluten free), light coconut milk
  - ❂ Dry milk powder: good way to add calcium and protein to your dishes
  - ❂ Sparkling water

Produce

- ❂ Vegetables (see chapter 4 for recommendations on when to buy organic vegetables and fruit):
  - ❂ Greens: baby spinach, kale, chard, arugula, Romaine lettuce, bagged salad (great convenience factor)
  - ❂ Onions, shallots, garlic, ginger
  - ❂ Carrots (consider pre-cut for convenient snacking), celery, bell peppers, broccoli, Brussels sprouts, cauliflower, sweet potatoes, butternut squash, avocado, cherry tomatoes, corn, green beans, cucumber, eggplant
- ❂ Fruits:
  - ❂ Apples, pears, oranges, clementines, grapefruit, bananas, grapes, stone fruit (plums, peaches, nectarines), melon, kiwi, lemons, limes
  - ❂ Berries (in season; frozen if out of season): strawberries, blueberries, raspberries, blackberries
- ❂ Fresh herbs: parsley, cilantro, mint, thyme, rosemary

Refrigerator
- ❀ Dairy:
  - ❀ Milk:
    - – Low-fat (1%) or reduced-fat (2%) milk: consider buying organic. Milk from organic, grass-fed cows is produced without antibiotics, hormones, or pesticides, and also provides higher amounts of omega-3 fatty acids
    - – Fortified almond or soy milk
  - ❀ Greek yogurt: reduced fat or low fat
  - ❀ Cheese: consider buying organic
    - – Shredded cheese like cheddar or mozzarella, string cheese or cheese sticks, crumbled pasteurized feta and goat cheese; Parmigiano-Reggiano or Pecorino Romano
    - – Cottage cheese, ricotta cheese, cream cheese (like reduced-fat Neufchâtel)
  - ❀ Unsalted butter
- ❀ Meat/Poultry/Seafood/Eggs/Soy Protein: consider buying organic for meat, poultry, and eggs. Organically raised animals are not given any antibiotics or hormones. Meat from grass-fed, organically raised cattle tends to be leaner and has higher levels of omega-3s. Don't bother buying organic for seafood as the USDA has not set the same standards for the labeling of seafood.
  - ❀ Fish: wild Atlantic salmon, cod, halibut, tilapia
  - ❀ Shrimp: buy shelled and deveined to save time (frozen is another good option)
  - ❀ Chicken breast: raw for cooking, and precooked strips to add to salads
  - ❀ Lean ground turkey and beef, turkey sausage
  - ❀ Lean cuts of beef (like flank steak), pork (like tenderloin) or other meat
  - ❀ Eggs: buy DHA-enhanced eggs, sometimes called omega-3 eggs. They're laid by chickens on a vegetarian, DHA-supplemented diet
  - ❀ Tofu: silken (for smoothies) and firm (for stir-fry); tempeh

❀ Other
  ❀ Juice: orange (calcium-fortified), pomegranate, vegetable juice
  ❀ Hummus
  ❀ Dijon mustard
  ❀ Mayonnaise (reduced fat)

Freezer

❀ Fruits and veggies are flash frozen at their peak to retain their nutrients and freshness
  ❀ Vegetables: mixed vegetables like peas and carrots, edamame (shelled for stir fries, in the pod for snacking)
  ❀ Fruits: berries (great for smoothies), fruit that's hard to find out of season like mango, peaches, and pineapple
❀ Brown rice (sold frozen, great time saver; you can also freeze your own)
❀ Dessert: all natural fruit popsicles (watch the sugar content), frozen yogurt, regular or reduced-fat ice cream
❀ Pizza dough (preferably whole wheat)
❀ Waffles (whole grain)
❀ Bagels and bread (whole grain)

Foods That Freeze Well

Meat, burgers, poultry, fish, bread, pizza dough, muffins, cakes, cookies, rice, butter, soups, stews, casseroles, chili, meatloaf, tomato sauce, tomato paste*, some fresh herbs*, pesto*

*freeze in ice cube trays for individual portions

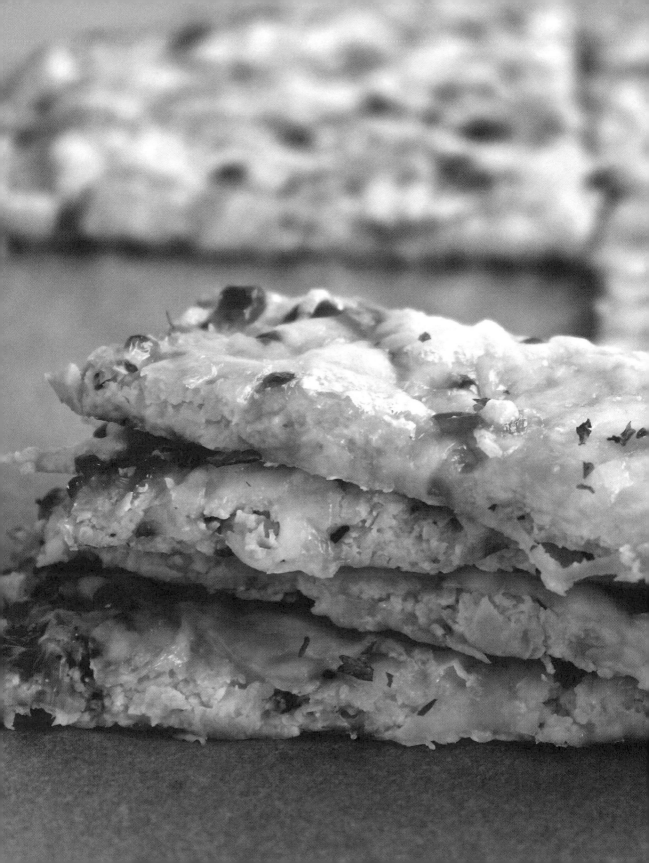

PART 2

THE RECIPES

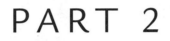

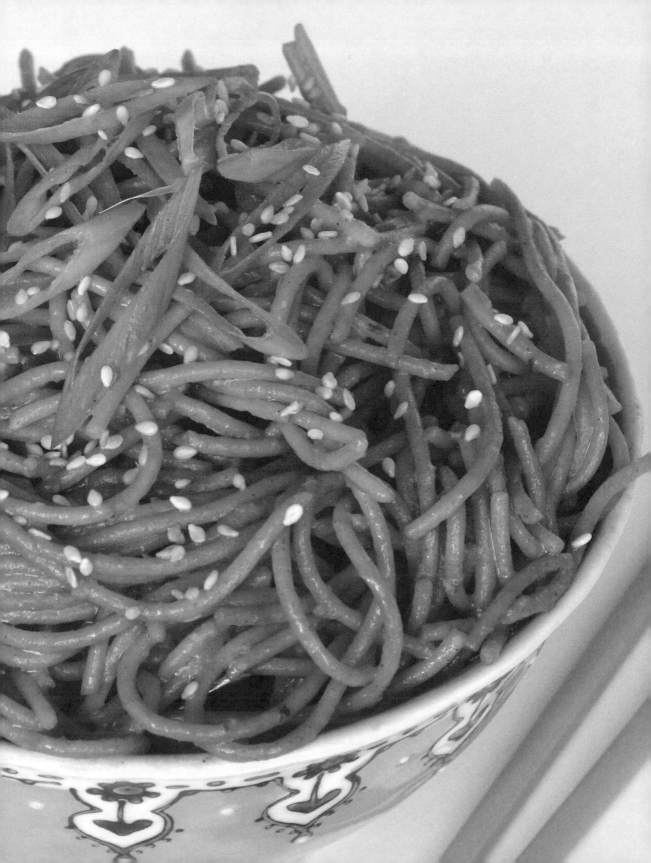

THIS SECTION WILL PROVIDE you with a wide range of delicious, healthy recipes suitable for a variety of tastes and preferences. Let's face it—your likes and dislikes evolve and change over time! I've spoken with a number of women who've experienced pregnancy firsthand, asking them for the kinds of recipes *they* would want to see in a cookbook for pregnant mothers. I asked them which foods they craved and which ones they couldn't stand. My goal was to provide plenty of mouthwatering recipes, enough to satisfy everyone's palate. For those days of intense cravings, I've included nutritious recipes that will satisfy any number of needs—salty, sweet, sour, or spicy. No need to send your loved ones out to the store for a late night pickle and ice cream run! Instead, try *Refrigerator Dill Pickles* (page 117) when you're craving something sour, or homemade *One-Ingredient Banana Ice Cream* (page 256) or *Super-Fast Peach Frozen Yogurt* (page 255) to satisfy your sweet tooth—both take only minutes to make!

On days when you're feeling green in the gills and can't keep much down, you may want to try a mild recipe, such as a smoothie; smoothies are easy on the stomach while still providing important nutrients. Feeling under the weather? Fight off that cold naturally by curling up with a bowl of *Classic Chicken Noodle Soup* (page 146) or another of my comforting soups. Tired of drinking plain water, but want to stay hydrated? I've included many delicious beverages that will quench your thirst and your cravings. I've even included some fun mocktails, so you don't have to feel left out at the party. Pregnant in the summertime? Beat the heat with one of my many refreshing cold treats like *Cherry Lime Granita* (page 260). Need quick recipe ideas that can be made in less than 30 minutes? No problem—try the *Quick and Easy Miso Glazed Salmon* (page 168). But perhaps you *want* to spend a leisurely day in the kitchen. My *Balsamic, Maple, and Thyme Roasted Chicken* (page 194) or *Sunday Beef Stew* (page 200) are the ultimate comfort foods. Looking to stock your freezer in preparation for your baby's arrival? Many of these dishes are freezer-friendly and can be stored for several months. You can have a home-cooked meal, even on days when you don't have the time or energy to cook.

For each recipe, I've provided a nutritional breakdown, helping you to keep track of what you're eating and letting you choose which recipes to make, based on your individual needs. I've also included several vegetarian recipes, with many others that can easily be adapted into vegetarian recipes.

Take a look through the recipes, find the ones that appeal to you the most, and get cooking!

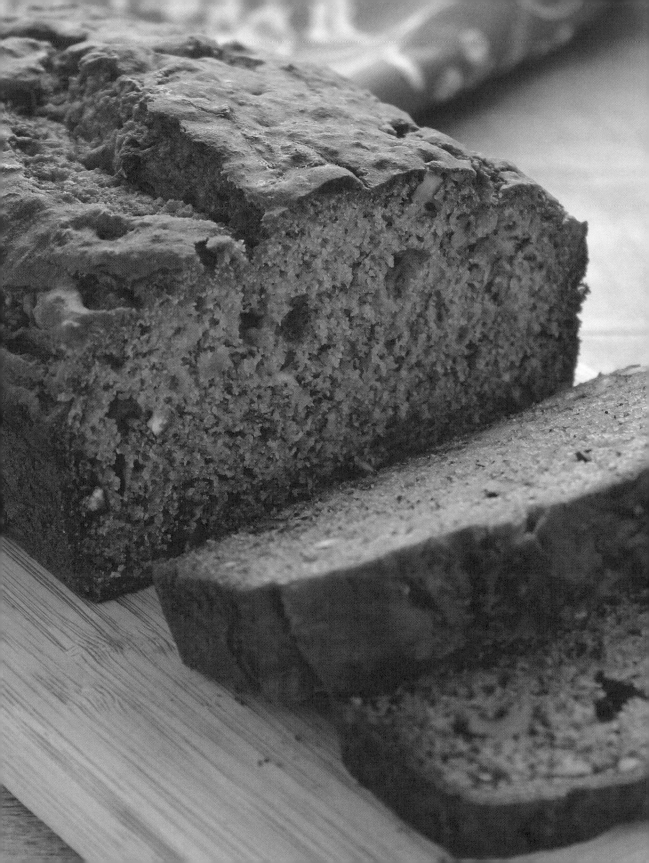

BREAKFAST

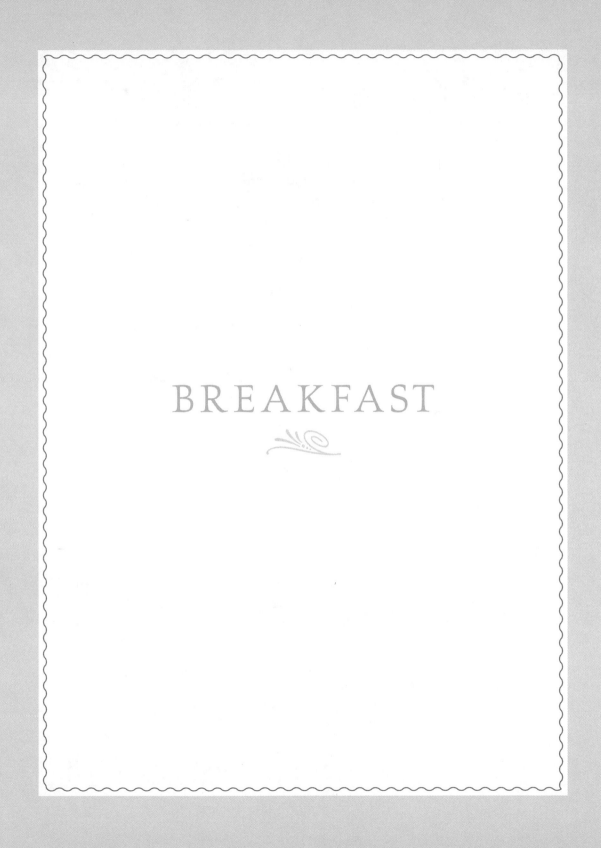

Rise and Shine Blueberry Oatmeal Muffins

MAKES 16 MUFFINS

Do yourself and your baby a favor and grab one of these delicious muffins on your way out the door in the morning! This portable breakfast is packed with plenty of whole grains, protein, fiber, antioxidants, vitamins, and minerals to fuel your day. I include wheat germ in the batter because it's a great source of folate and zinc, both of which are crucial for your baby's development. These muffins freeze well so make a whole batch and pop them in the microwave in the morning or anytime you want a quick snack.

¾ cup enriched all-purpose flour
¾ cup white whole wheat flour
1½ cups quick-cooking oats
½ cup wheat germ
¾ cup coconut palm sugar or light
   brown sugar
2 teaspoons baking soda
½ teaspoon baking powder
1½ teaspoons cinnamon

½ teaspoon kosher salt
1 large egg
1 cup reduced-fat vanilla Greek
   yogurt
½ cup low-fat milk
⅓ cup safflower or other neutral-
   flavored oil
1½ cups blueberries (fresh or frozen)

Preheat oven to 375°F. Line two 12-cup muffin tins with 16 paper muffin liners.

Mix the flours, oats, wheat germ, sugar, baking soda, baking powder, cinnamon and salt together in a large mixing bowl. Mix the egg, yogurt, milk, and oil in a second bowl. Add the wet ingredients to the dry ingredients and stir until just combined (do not over-mix). Gently stir the blueberries into the batter.

Scoop the batter into the muffin cups and fill them about ¾ of the way full (you should have 16 muffins). Bake 18 to 20 minutes until muffins are golden brown and a toothpick inserted into the center comes out clean. Cool in the pan for 5 to 10 minutes and then turn the muffins onto a rack and cool completely. Muffins can be served right away, refrigerated, or frozen for later use.

NUTRITIONAL INFORMATION
One muffin: Calories 206; Fat 6.4g (Sat 0.9g); Protein 6.2g; Carb 31.6g; Fiber 3.3g; Calcium 65mg; Iron 1.6mg; Sodium 265mg; Folate 42mg

Quick-cooking oats are the same as rolled or old-fashioned oats save that they are coarsely chopped so that they cook faster. If you only have rolled oats, you can give them a quick whir in the food processor to make quick-cooking oats. Use about 1¾ cup rolled oats to yield 1½ cups quick-cooking oats.

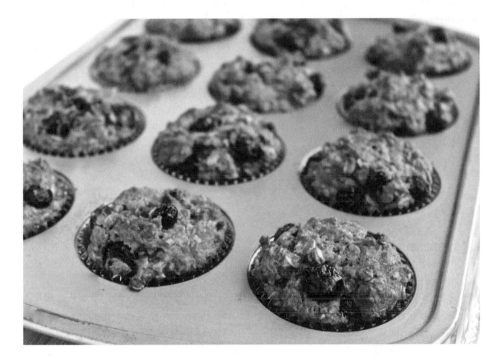

"Pump Up Your Milk" Pumpkin Chocolate Chip Muffins

MAKES ABOUT 18 MUFFINS

This recipe was shared by my friend and fellow blogger Justine. She and her sister have a wonderful site called Full Belly Sisters (www.fullbellysisters.blogspot.com), which offers useful tools to help women stay healthy and informed while they're pregnant, breastfeeding, or just striving for balance in their lives. Justine notes that the chia seeds, flaxseed and brewer's yeast are optional in this recipe but recommended if you're breastfeeding, as they add omega-3s, protein, fiber, calcium, and B vitamins. Additionally, both flax and brewer's yeast may help support a healthy milk supply.

2 eggs

½ cup honey

1 cup pureed pumpkin

½ cup (melted) coconut or grapeseed oil

½ cup unsweetened applesauce

1 teaspoon vanilla

1 cup whole wheat flour

⅔ cup almond flour

1 teaspoon baking soda

½ teaspoon salt

½ teaspoon baking powder

½ cup chopped walnuts

⅓ cup chocolate chips + extra to top muffins (or dried fruit like raisins or cranberries)

2 tablespoons chia seeds (optional)

3 tablespoons flaxseed meal (optional)

2 tablespoons brewer's yeast (optional)

Preheat oven to 350°F. Whisk together the wet ingredients (eggs through vanilla). In another bowl, combine the dry ingredients (whole wheat flour through brewer's yeast). Add the dry ingredients to the wet and mix well.

Line muffin tins with paper. Fill each to the top with batter and top each with a chocolate chip (optional). Bake 25 to 30 minutes for regular muffins, 22 minutes for mini muffins, and 55 minutes for a loaf. They are ready when a toothpick inserted in the middle comes out clean.

Cool for a few minutes in the pan on a rack. Then, remove from the pan and cool completely on a rack.

NUTRITIONAL INFORMATION

One muffin: Calories 196; Fat 12.1g (Sat 1.8g); Protein 4.6g; Carb 19g; Fiber 2.9g; Calcium 31mg; Iron 1mg; Sodium 231mg; Folate 30mg

Baby Bump Banana Flax Bread

MAKES 12 SERVINGS

Who doesn't love a good banana bread? This banana bread not only tastes great, it also provides several important nutrients to nourish both you and your growing baby. I use a mixture of white whole wheat and all-purpose flour to incorporate nutritious whole grains. Flaxseed provides brain-boosting omega-3s, and Greek yogurt bumps up the protein and calcium content. I also like to add heart-healthy nuts like pecans or walnuts, but if you have a nut allergy or are just not a fan, you can leave them out (or substitute dark chocolate chips). For this recipe, you'll want to use the ripest bananas possible. It's a great way to use up the ones that are sitting on your counter getting brown!

1½ cups mashed, very ripe bananas (3 or 4 bananas)
⅓ cup reduced-fat vanilla Greek yogurt
2 large eggs
¼ cup safflower oil (or other neutral-flavored oil)
½ teaspoon vanilla
⅔ cup coconut palm sugar or light brown sugar

¾ cup enriched all-purpose flour
¾ cup white whole wheat flour
⅓ cup ground flaxseed
1½ teaspoons baking soda
½ teaspoon cinnamon
¼ teaspoon salt
½ cup chopped pecans or walnuts (optional)

Preheat oven to 350°F. Mix the bananas, yogurt, egg, oil, and vanilla together in the bowl of a stand mixer until combined. Add the sugar and continue to mix until combined.

Whisk the flours, flaxseed, baking soda, cinnamon, and salt together in a medium bowl. Add the dry ingredients to the wet ingredients in the mixer and beat until just combined (do not over-mix). Stir the nuts into the batter.

Pour the batter into a 9 x 5-inch loaf pan coated with cooking spray. Bake in the oven for 50 to 55 minutes, or until a toothpick inserted into the center comes out clean. Remove from oven and cool for 10 minutes in the pan on a wire rack. Remove the bread and cool completely on wire rack.

NUTRITIONAL INFORMATION
One serving: Calories 224; Fat 10.5g (Sat 1.2g); Protein 4.8g; Carb 28.8g; Fiber 3.5g; Calcium 44mg; Iron 1.3mg; Sodium 225mg; Folate 41mg

Apple Cinnamon Dutch Baby

MAKES 4 SERVINGS

I couldn't resist including a recipe with the word "baby" in the name! A Dutch baby, also called a German pancake, is a baked breakfast dish that's like a cross between a popover and a pancake. It's traditionally baked in the oven in a cast-iron skillet and has a delightfully light, tender, eggy interior with crispy edges. Serve it straight from the oven with a dusting of powdered sugar while it's still puffed up high. This dish will provide you with a good amount of calcium, protein, folate, and choline. Using a cast-iron skillet will also help boost your iron.

2 tablespoons unsalted butter, divided
1 large apple, thinly sliced
2 tablespoons light brown sugar, divided
½ teaspoon cinnamon
3 large eggs at room temperature

¾ cup low-fat milk, warm
¾ cup enriched all-purpose flour
½ teaspoon vanilla extract
¼ teaspoon salt
1 teaspoon powdered sugar
Maple syrup for serving (optional)

Preheat oven to 400°F. Heat 1 tablespoon butter over medium heat in a 10-inch oven-safe skillet (preferably cast-iron). When the butter is melted, add the apples, 1 tablespoon light brown sugar, and cinnamon. Stir to combine. Cook until apples start to soften, about 4 to 5 minutes.

While the apples cook, melt the remaining tablespoon butter in the microwave. Pour it into a blender along with the eggs, milk, flour, vanilla, salt, and remaining 1 tablespoon of sugar. Blend until smooth. Alternatively you can whisk the eggs and milk together in a bowl until blended and light yellow. Then whisk in the flour, vanilla, salt, and sugar until smooth.

Pour the batter over the apples in the skillet and transfer the skillet to the oven. Bake 20 to 25 minutes until puffed up and golden brown. Dust with powdered sugar and serve with maple syrup, if desired. Serve immediately, as it will start to fall within minutes of being taken out of the oven.

NUTRITIONAL INFORMATION
One serving: Calories 261; Fat 9.3g (Sat 5.2g); Protein 9.2g; Carb 33.8g; Fiber 2.1g; Calcium 101mg; Iron 1.9mg; Sodium 228mg; Folate 89µg

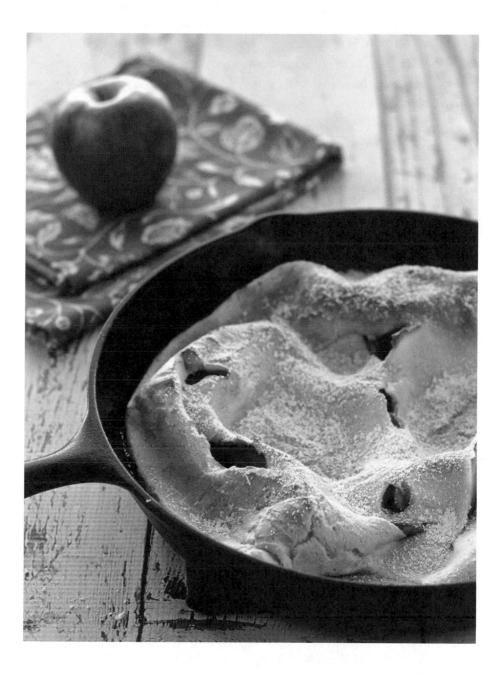

Berry and Ricotta Stuffed French Toast

MAKES 4 SERVINGS

Get pampered with this stuffed French toast that's perfect for breakfast in bed. You'll want to dive right into this luxurious and deceptively healthy breakfast treat. Sweet berry jam is mixed with creamy ricotta cheese and sandwiched between layers of whole grain bread before being bathed in an eggy batter and crisped to perfection. Who would think that it's also packed with protein, fiber, and loads of calcium to get your day going?

¾ cup part-skim ricotta cheese
3 tablespoons berry jam or preserves
    (can use Blackberry Chia Jam on
    page 87)
8 slices whole grain bread
2 cup mixed berries such as
    blueberries, raspberries,
    blackberries, and sliced
    strawberries, divided

3 large eggs
⅔ cup skim or low-fat milk
1 teaspoon vanilla
2 teaspoons olive oil
2 teaspoons butter
Optional toppings: powdered sugar,
    maple syrup or Blueberry Maple
    Compote (page 87)

Mix the ricotta and jam together in a bowl. Spread equal amounts of the mixture on four pieces of bread. Sprinkle ¼ cup berries on top of each piece of bread (reserve the rest of the berries for the topping). Place the remaining four pieces of bread on top to form four sandwiches.

Beat the eggs, milk, and vanilla together in baking dish or other wide, shallow dish.

Heat the oil and butter in a large skillet over medium heat. Carefully dip each sandwich into the egg mixture until completely moistened, then flip and soak the other side. Remove the sandwiches from the egg mixture and cook them in the skillet, about 3 to 4 minutes on each side, until golden brown.

Transfer to serving plates. Cut each sandwich in half on a diagonal and sprinkle the remaining berries around the plate. Top with desired toppings like powdered sugar, maple syrup, or Blueberry Maple Compote (see page 87).

NUTRITIONAL INFORMATION
One serving: Calories 383; Fat 12.2g (Sat 5.3g); Protein 18.7g; Carb 48.8g; Fiber 5.6g; Calcium 260mg; Iron 2.5mg; Sodium 391mg; Folate 57mg

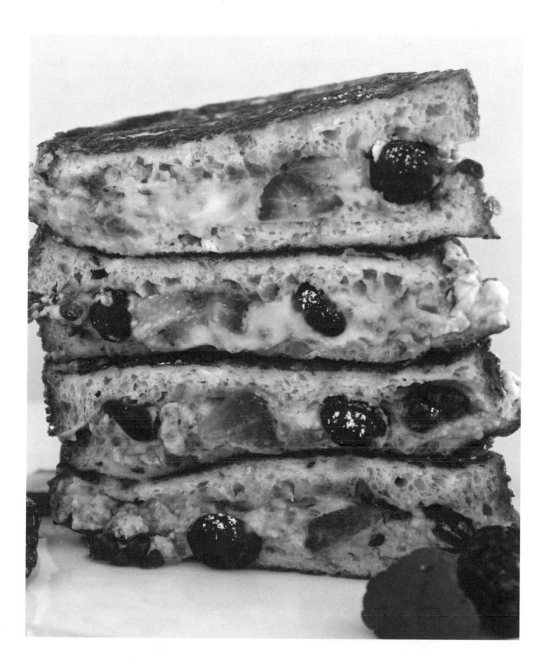

good → more lemon zest is good!

Lemon Ricotta Blueberry Pancakes

MAKES 12 PANCAKES OR 6 SERVINGS

The next time you want to enjoy a leisurely breakfast, try making these pancakes that are bursting with bright, lemony flavor. Studded with vibrant blueberries, this dish will supply you with whole grains, calcium, folate, and fiber. Ricotta cheese makes the pancakes tender and adds a boost of protein to keep you feeling full. The secret to keeping these pancakes light and fluffy is to fold whipped egg whites into the batter at the end.

¾ cup white whole wheat flour
¾ cup all-purpose flour
1 teaspoon baking soda
½ teaspoon kosher salt
2 large eggs, yolks and whites separated
1¼ cups reduced-fat buttermilk
2 tablespoons sugar

2 tablespoons lemon juice
1 tablespoon lemon zest
½ cup ricotta cheese
6 ounces blueberries
Optional toppings: maple syrup or Blueberry Maple Compote (page 87)

Whisk both types of flour, baking soda, and salt together in a small bowl. Whisk the egg yolks, buttermilk, sugar, lemon juice, lemon zest, and ricotta cheese together in a large bowl. Place the egg whites in the bowl of a stand mixer and beat them until soft peaks form. Alternatively, you can use a hand held mixer to beat the egg whites.

Stir the dry ingredients into the bowl with the wet ingredients until just combined (do not over-mix). Gently fold the egg whites into the batter until they are incorporated. The batter will be thick.

Heat a large nonstick pan or griddle over medium heat and coat with cooking spray. Using a ¼ cup measure, spoon the batter into the pan in batches. Scatter some blueberries on each pancake.

Cook until the pancakes start to bubble around the edges and get lightly browned, about 2 to 3 minutes. Flip and cook until golden brown on the other side, about 2 to 3 minutes more. Remove from heat and serve immediately. Alternatively, you may place the pancakes on a baking sheet in the oven at 200°F to keep them warm until all of them are cooked. Serve pancakes with maple syrup, if desired. Garnish with remaining blueberries and lemon zest.

NUTRITIONAL INFORMATION
One serving (2 pancakes): Calories 229; Fat 5.4g (Sat 3g); Protein 10.3g; Carb 35g; Fiber 2.8g; Calcium 135mg; Iron 1.8mg; Sodium 488mg; Folate 67μg

---

Turkey Sausage Egg White Flatbread

MAKES 4 SANDWICHES

My friend Carrie over at Carrie's Experimental Kitchen (www.carriesexperimental kitchen.com) created these yummy breakfast sandwiches as an alternative to the egg sandwiches she used to buy at a coffee shop. By using fresh, whole ingredients, she was able to make a much healthier dish with fewer calories, less fat, sodium, sugar, and other additives. I love these sandwiches because you can make a large batch and freeze them. Then, before you head out the door in the morning, you can heat one up and have a nutritious breakfast in minutes! This dish is a good source of protein, fiber, and calcium and will give you the energy you need to get your day going. Baking the eggs in a muffin tin is an easy way to make perfect eggs every time.

2 links cooked breakfast turkey
    sausage, diced small
¼ cup chopped, fresh spinach
8 large egg whites

4 multigrain sandwich rounds
4 slices ultra-thin mild cheddar
    cheese

Preheat oven to 350°F. In a medium bowl, combine the turkey sausage, spinach, and egg whites. Mix well.

Spray a muffin top pan with olive oil cooking spray and spoon the mixture into four of the cups. Alternatively, you can use a 6-cup jumbo muffin pan. Bake for 15 minutes or until the tops bounce back when touched. If using a jumbo muffin pan, bake for 22 to 25 minutes.

Remove the eggs from the pan and place each one on the bottom of a sandwich round. Top each with a slice of cheese and the sandwich round tops. Serve immediately or wrap tightly in aluminum foil and freeze for later use.

NUTRITIONAL INFORMATION
One serving: Calories 199; Fat 5.3g (Sat 2.5g); Protein 16.6g; Carb 19.7g; Fiber 4g; Calcium 129mg; Iron 1.4mg; Sodium 431mg; Folate 40µg

---

Note: To reheat frozen sandwiches, let them defrost naturally in the fridge overnight or place them in the oven or toaster oven. You can also reheat them in the microwave. To do this, remove the foil and wrap the sandwiches in paper towels before heating.

Summer Zucchini and Corn Frittata

MAKES 4 SERVINGS

A frittata is an Italian egg dish similar to an omelet but less complicated. No fancy flipping techniques involved here—simply sauté your ingredients in a skillet and then pop it in the oven to finish cooking. I like to mix some Greek yogurt into the eggs because it adds a boost of protein and also gives the finished dish a nice, fluffy texture. This frittata uses zucchini and corn, two of my favorite summer vegetables, but the great thing about frittatas is that you can use whatever ingredients you have in your fridge or pantry. Although traditionally served for breakfast, frittatas are perfect for quick weeknight dinners as well. This nutritious dish is rich in protein, calcium, folate, and choline.

2 teaspoons olive oil
2 medium zucchini, very thinly sliced (preferably on a mandoline)
2 cloves garlic, minced
1 cup fresh corn kernels (can use frozen)
8 eggs
¼ cup nonfat Greek yogurt

⅛ teaspoon cayenne pepper
½ teaspoon salt
¼ teaspoon black pepper
1 ounce grated Parmigiano-Reggiano cheese (about ¼ cup)
2 tablespoons chopped, fresh parsley for garnish

Preheat oven to 400°F. Heat the oil in a medium ovenproof skillet (preferably cast-iron) over medium heat. Add the zucchini and cook, stirring occasionally, until it starts to soften, about 5 to 6 minutes. Add the garlic and corn and cook another 3 to 4 minutes until tender.

In a bowl, whisk the eggs, Greek yogurt, cayenne, salt, and pepper. Pour the mixture into the skillet with the vegetables. Cook for a few minutes until the edges start to set. As it cooks, gently push the edges towards the middle with a spatula allowing the liquid to come into contact with the bottom of the skillet.

Sprinkle the cheese evenly over the top of the eggs and place the skillet in the oven. Bake 8 to 10 minutes until the frittata is fully cooked and puffed up. For a golden brown color, turn the broiler on and cook another 2 to 3 minutes until the top is browned. Remove from oven, garnish with parsley and serve.

NUTRITIONAL INFORMATION
One serving: Calories 234; Fat 12.5g (Sat 4.5g); Protein 17.8g; Carb 12g; Fiber 1.9g; Calcium 179mg; Iron 2.4mg; Sodium 542mg; Folate 84µg

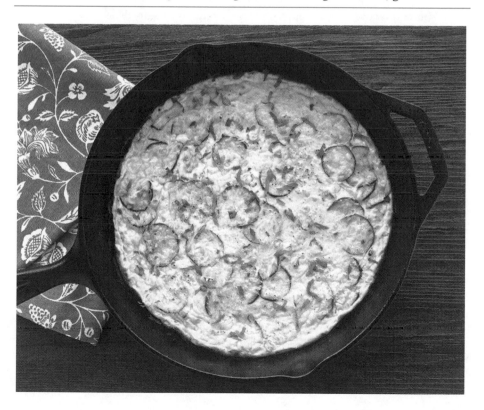

Spinach, Mushroom, and Gruyere Breakfast Strata

MAKES 8 SERVINGS

This is a perfect dish for Sunday brunch. A strata is a layered casserole made with cubed bread, eggs, cheese, and other ingredients, like vegetables or meat. It's similar to a savory bread pudding and it's definitely a comfort food. The beauty in making strata is that you can prepare it all the night before and in the morning, simply bake it and serve it straight out of the oven while it's puffed up. Day-old or stale bread works best to soak up the custard. You can also bake individual portions of the mixture in a muffin pan for a convenient and healthy grab-and-go breakfast. This recipe is packed with protein and calcium. It's also a good source of fiber, folate, and iron.

10 ounces day-old or stale multi-grain (whole grain) bread cut into ¾-inch pieces (about 8 cups)

1½ tablespoons olive oil

¼ cup chopped shallots

10 ounces cremini mushrooms, sliced

1 box (10 ounces) frozen, chopped spinach, defrosted and squeezed dry

¾ teaspoon dried thyme (or 1 tablespoon fresh)

1 teaspoon salt, divided

½ teaspoon pepper, divided

8 large eggs

2 cups low-fat milk

1 tablespoon Dijon mustard

3 ounces grated Gruyere cheese, divided

Place the bread in a large bowl. Heat the oil in a large skillet over medium heat. Add the shallots and cook for 1 to 2 minutes, until tender. Add the mushrooms and cook for 3 to 4 minutes until they start to soften. Add the spinach and stir to combine. Season the mixture with the thyme, ½ teaspoon salt, and ¼ teaspoon pepper. Transfer the mixture to the bowl with the bread and mix the ingredients together.

Whisk the eggs, milk, mustard, ½ teaspoon salt, ¼ teaspoon pepper, and about ¾ of the cheese together in another bowl.

Spray an 8 x 12-inch baking dish with cooking spray. Transfer the bread and vegetable mixture to the dish, spreading it out evenly. Pour the egg mixture over the top and gently press the bread down into the liquid. Sprinkle the remaining cheese on top. Alternatively, to make individual portions, divide the mixture between the cups of a muffin pan (it will make about 16 portions, so you may need two pans).

Let the mixture sit while you preheat the oven to 350°F. Alternatively, the dish can be prepared the night before and allowed to soak in the refrigerator overnight. Bake strata in the oven uncovered for 50 to 60 minutes (30 to 40 minutes if using a muffin pan) until it is puffed up and golden brown. Cut into pieces and serve.

NUTRITIONAL INFORMATION
One serving: Calories 286; Fat 12.3g (Sat 4.7g); Protein 19.1g; Carb 22.8g; Fiber 4.1g; Calcium 310mg; Iron 2.9mg; Sodium 542mg; Folate 113μg

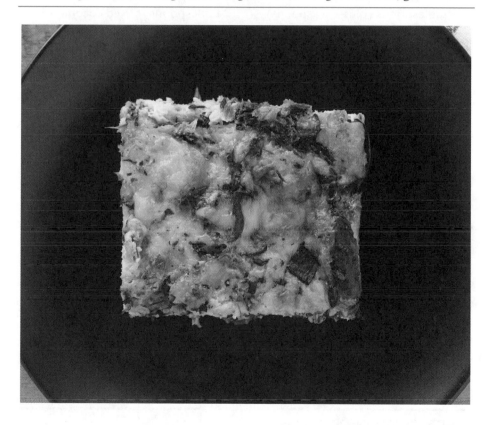

Peachy-Keen Baked Oatmeal

MAKES 6 SERVINGS

If you've never experienced the wonders of baked oatmeal, you must try this recipe! Oats and fresh peaches are baked together in a hearty and comforting breakfast dish that tastes so good it almost feels like dessert. This dish is a good source of whole grains, protein, fiber, calcium, and iron. Feel free to use different fruits if you don't like peaches—fresh berries and bananas are wonderful choices. Serve it alone or topped with maple syrup, milk, or Greek yogurt.

2 cups rolled oats
¼ cup sliced almonds
2 tablespoons (plus 2 teaspoons) coconut palm sugar or brown sugar, divided
1 teaspoon baking powder
½ teaspoon cinnamon plus extra for garnish
¼ teaspoon salt
2 cups low-fat milk or unsweetened almond milk

1 large egg
2 tablespoons maple syrup
2 tablespoons melted coconut oil or unsalted butter
1 teaspoon vanilla extract
12 ounces (about 2 cups) diced peaches plus a few slices of peaches for garnish

Preheat oven to 350°F. Spray an 8 x 8-inch baking dish with cooking spray. Mix the oats, almonds, 2 tablespoons sugar, baking powder, cinnamon, and salt together in a medium bowl. Whisk the milk, egg, maple syrup, coconut oil, and vanilla together in another bowl.

Scatter the diced peaches in the bottom of the prepared baking dish. Pour the oat mixture evenly on top. Pour the milk mixture on top and press to submerge all of the dry ingredients in the liquid. Arrange the peach slices on top and sprinkle with the remaining 2 teaspoons sugar and a pinch of cinnamon.

Bake for 35 to 40 minutes, until set. Let rest for 10 minutes before serving. Serve the oatmeal alone or top with a little milk, maple syrup, or vanilla Greek yogurt.

NUTRITIONAL INFORMATION
One serving: Calories 371; Fat 10.8g (Sat 5.6g); Protein 14.4g; Carb 54.2g; Fiber 7g; Calcium 219mg; Iron 3.1mg; Sodium 240mg; Folate 41mg

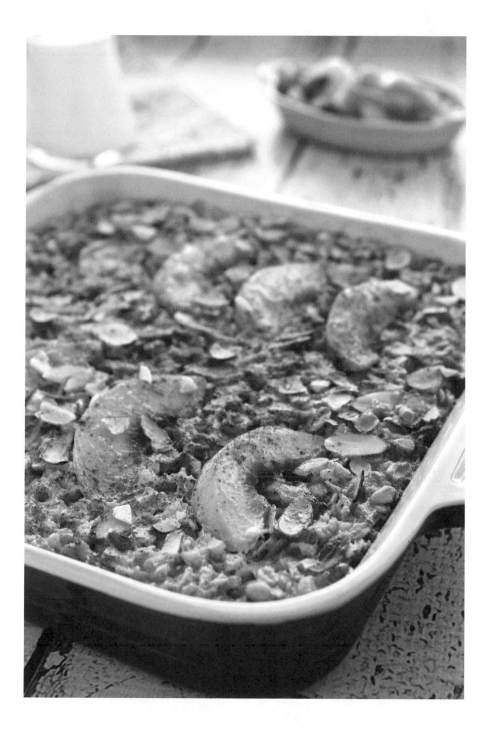

Coconut Maple Granola

MAKES ABOUT 3½ CUPS

Did you know that making your own granola at home is really easy? It's also healthier than buying it at the store as many brands contain hidden sugar and fat. This granola packs a fiber punch with oats, nuts, seeds, and dried fruit. It makes a great snack and will help prevent constipation when your intestinal tract slows down. You can also enjoy it with milk or yogurt for a well-balanced breakfast.

2 cups rolled oats
½ cup shredded unsweetened
   coconut
¼ cup sliced almonds
¼ cup chopped pecans
¼ cup sunflower seeds
½ teaspoon cinnamon
¼ teaspoon kosher salt

3 tablespoons safflower or coconut
   oil
2 tablespoons maple syrup
2 tablespoons brown sugar
1 teaspoon vanilla extract
⅓ cup reduced sugar dried
   cranberries or other dried fruit

Preheat oven to 300°F. Mix the oats, coconut, almonds, pecans, sunflower seeds, cinnamon, and salt together in a large bowl.

In a small saucepan, heat the oil, maple syrup, and sugar together. Once melted, remove from heat and stir in the vanilla extract. Pour into the oat mixture and stir until well coated.

Spread the granola out in a thin layer on a baking sheet lined with a silicone baking mat. Bake in the oven for about 25 to 30 minutes, stirring the granola once or twice. Remove the tray from the oven and stir in the dried cranberries. Allow the granola to cool completely (it will crisp up as it cools).

Serve the granola plain or with milk or yogurt. Store in an airtight container in the refrigerator.

NUTRITIONAL INFORMATION
One serving (¼ cup): Calories 194; Fat 9.3g (Sat 2.5g); Protein 4.9g; Carb 23.5g; Fiber 4.5g; Calcium 25mg; Iron 1.5mg; Sodium 43mg; Folate 19µg

Blueberry Maple Compote

MAKES 1 CUP

This quick and easy compote is the perfect accompaniment to Berry and Ricotta Stuffed French Toast (page 76) and Lemon Ricotta Blueberry Pancakes (page 78). Try it as an alternative to plain maple syrup. The blueberries add powerful disease-fighting antioxidants as well as Vitamin C, Vitamin K, and fiber.

1½ cups blueberries
3 tablespoons pure maple syrup
⅛ teaspoon cinnamon

Place all of the ingredients in a small saucepan and bring to a boil. Reduce heat to a simmer and cook for 5 minutes, until the blueberries start to break down. Crush some of the berries lightly with a fork. Let the compote cool slightly before serving. Serve compote with French toast or pancakes.

NUTRITIONAL INFORMATION
One serving (¼ cup): Calories 70; Fat 0.1g (Sat 0g); Protein 0.4g; Carb 18.2g; Fiber 1.4g; Calcium 19mg; Iron 0.2mg; Sodium 2mg; Folate 3mg

Blackberry Chia Jam

MAKES ABOUT 1½ CUPS

Cha-cha-cha-chia! Who would have thought that the novelty plant from the 80s would turn out to be a super food with amazing health benefits? Chia seeds are packed with omega-3 fatty acids, antioxidants, fiber, protein, calcium, and several other nutrients. In addition, these powerful little seeds absorb water and have an amazing gelling property. When they're added to fresh-cooked berries, the mixture thickens up to make an easy and nutritious jam.

1 pound fresh blackberries
   (can substitute blueberries,
   strawberries, or raspberries)

1 tablespoon lemon juice
¼ cup maple syrup
3 tablespoons chia seeds

Heat the blackberries in a saucepan over medium heat. Simmer for 6 to 7 minutes until the berries start to soften and break down. Mash the berries lightly with a potato masher or fork, leaving some chunks. Stir in the lemon juice, maple syrup, and chia seeds and cook for a few more minutes, stirring often. Turn the heat off and let the mixture cool. As it cools, the jam will thicken. Store jam in an airtight container in the refrigerator for up to 2 weeks.

NUTRITIONAL INFORMATION
One serving (2 tablespoons): Calories 46; Fat 0.9g (Sat 0.1g); Protein 1g; Carb 9.3g; Fiber 3g; Calcium 34mg; Iron 0.2mg; Sodium 1mg; Folate 9µg

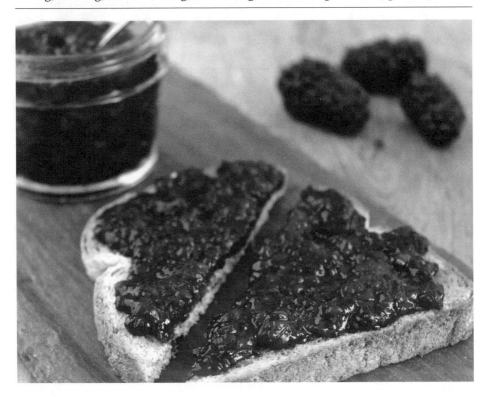

Sunshiny Day Breakfast Parfaits

MAKES 4 SERVINGS

You eat this dish with your eyes first—when you see these beautiful breakfast parfaits, you'll want to dive right in! Layers of Greek yogurt are swirled with fresh homemade jam and topped with crunchy granola and sweet berries. This nutritious breakfast dish will provide you with plenty of calcium, protein, fiber, and antioxidants to get your day going. Chia seeds also supply a good amount of healthy omega-3s. This recipe calls for my Blackberry Chia Jam (page 87) and Coconut Maple Granola, (page 86) but you can substitute these with store-bought fruit jam and granola if you're short on time. Just check the nutrition labels though, as many of these products are high in added sugars.

3 cups reduced-fat plain Greek yogurt

½ cup Blackberry Chia Jam (recipe on page 87)

½ cup Coconut Maple Granola (recipe on page 86)

1 cup fresh berries (e.g., blueberries, blackberries, raspberries, or strawberries)

Place ½ cup yogurt in the bottom of each of four bowls or glasses. Spoon 2 tablespoons of the jam on top and swirl it into the yogurt. Sprinkle 2 tablespoons granola on top. Top with another ¼ cup yogurt and ¼ cup berries. Serve immediately.

NUTRITIONAL INFORMATION
One serving: Calories 309; Fat 10.7g (Sat 5.5g); Protein 21.1g; Carb 33.6g; Fiber 6.6g; Calcium 384mg; Iron 1.3mg; Sodium 79mg; Folate 40µg

Strawberry Almond Breakfast Quinoa

MAKES 4 SERVINGS

Start your day off right with this nutritious, whole grain breakfast. Quinoa is an ancient grain with spectacular health benefits. It's packed with protein, fiber, vitamins, and minerals—no wonder the Incas referred to it as the Mother Grain! Cook it in milk and top it with your favorite toppings for a filling breakfast that will jump-start your day. I use almond milk in this recipe but you can use regular milk, soy or rice milk—most varieties are fortified with calcium and Vitamin D to help your baby's bones grow strong.

1 cup quinoa, rinsed

2 cups (plus 2 tablespoons) unsweetened almond milk, divided

2 tablespoons pure maple syrup

¼ teaspoon cinnamon

1 cup sliced strawberries

2 tablespoons sliced almonds, toasted

2 tablespoons shredded, unsweetened coconut

Place the quinoa and 2 cups almond milk in a medium saucepan and bring to a boil. Lowering the heat to a simmer, cover the pot and cook, stirring occasionally, until quinoa is done (about 10 to 15 minutes). Stir in the remaining 2 tablespoons milk, maple syrup, and cinnamon.

Divide the quinoa among four bowls and top with equal portions of strawberries, almonds, and coconut. Serve immediately.

NUTRITIONAL INFORMATION
One serving: Calories 240; Fat 6.3g (Sat 1.5g); Protein 7.6g; Carb 38.4g; Fiber 4.6g; Calcium 270mg; Iron 2.5mg; Sodium 88mg; Folate 89µg

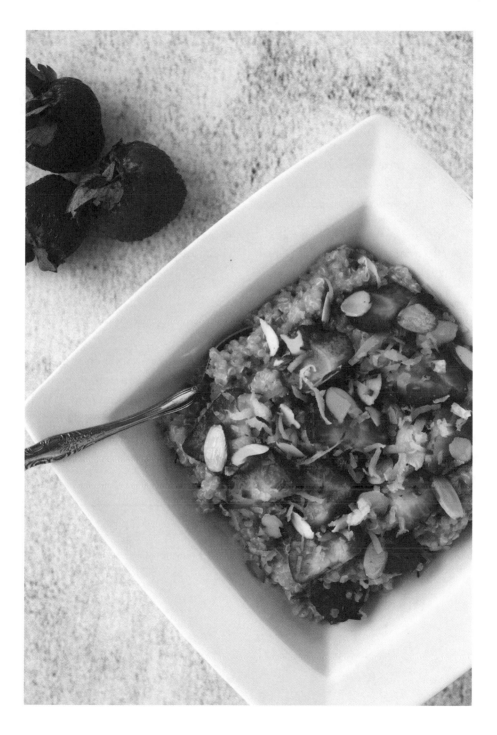

Almond Chia Pudding with Raspberries

MAKES 2 SERVINGS

What can be easier than mixing a few ingredients in a jar and letting it sit in the fridge overnight while you get your beauty sleep? Adding chia seeds to almond milk and yogurt thickens it up and turns it into a protein-packed pudding without much effort. These tiny seeds are packed with healthful nutrients that are beneficial for you and your little one. Chia is one of the most concentrated sources of omega-3 fatty acids, helping to boost the development of your baby's brain and eyes.

¾ cup unsweetened almond milk
¾ cup nonfat or low-fat plain Greek
   yogurt
3 tablespoons chia seeds
2 tablespoons maple syrup, honey,
   or sweetener of your choice

½ teaspoon vanilla extract
½ cup raspberries
Optional topping: sliced almonds

Place the almond milk, yogurt, chia seeds, maple syrup, and vanilla in a bowl and stir until combined. Alternatively you can pour the ingredients into a mason jar or other container with a lid and shake until ingredients are combined. Let the mixture sit for 15 to 20 minutes (the seeds will sink to the bottom), then stir it again. Place the container in the refrigerator and cool overnight. The mixture will thicken. When ready to serve, divide the pudding into two bowls and garnish with raspberries and almonds.

NUTRITIONAL INFORMATION
One serving: Calories 210; Fat 6g (Sat 0.5g); Protein 11.9g; Carb 27.3g; Fiber 8g; Calcium 466mg; Iron 0.5mg; Sodium 95mg; Folate 6µg

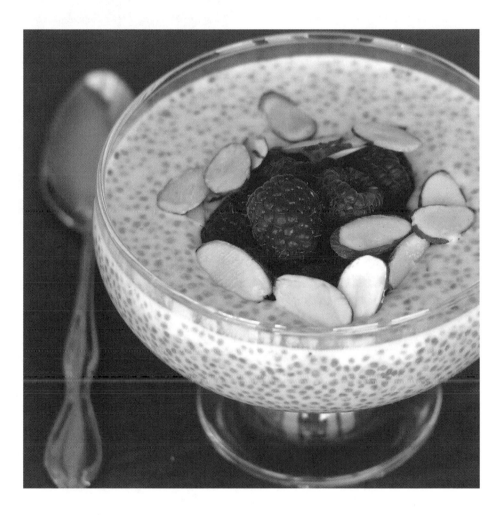

Blueberry Vanilla No-Cook Overnight Oats

EACH MAKES 1 SERVING

No time to make breakfast in the morning? No problem, you can make it the night before! Oats are nutritious whole grains and the great thing about them is that they don't even need to be cooked. Simply mix them with your favorite milk and stir in any number of other ingredients like fruits, nuts, seeds, or yogurt. Refrigerate overnight and in the morning, you'll have a hearty and nutritious breakfast waiting for you that's packed with protein, fiber, calcium, and iron. On the following pages are three variations—feel free to experiment and make your own unique creations.

⅓ cup low-fat milk or almond milk
⅓ cup low-fat vanilla Greek yogurt
⅓ cup rolled oats
½ teaspoon lemon juice

1 teaspoon chia seeds
½ cup fresh or frozen blueberries
1 tablespoon sliced almonds,
   toasted

Stir all ingredients except the almonds together in a mason jar or bowl. Cover and refrigerate overnight. In the morning, top with almonds and enjoy.

NUTRITIONAL INFORMATION
One serving: Calories 378; Fat 8g (Sat 1.7g); Protein 19g; Carb 59g; Fiber 9.3g; Calcium 347mg; Iron 3mg; Sodium 110mg; Folate 48µg

Nutty Nana No-Cook Overnight Oats

½ cup unsweetened vanilla
  almond milk or low-fat milk
1 tablespoon natural peanut
  butter
1 teaspoon honey (adjust to
  taste)

⅛ teaspoon cinnamon plus extra
  for garnish
½ cup rolled oats
1 teaspoon chia seeds
½ banana, chopped

Whisk the milk, peanut butter, honey, and cinnamon together in a bowl until smooth. Stir in the oats, chia seeds, and banana. Cover and refrigerate overnight. In the morning, sprinkle with cinnamon and enjoy.

NUTRITIONAL INFORMATION
One serving: Calories 502; Fat 14.7g (Sat 2.8g); Protein 18.9g; Carb 76g; Fiber 12.3g; Calcium 300mg; Iron 4.4mg; Sodium 83mg; Folate 65µg

Almond Joy No-Cook Overnight Oats

½ cup dark chocolate almond
  milk
½ cup rolled oats
1 teaspoon chia seeds

1 tablespoon sliced almonds,
  toasted
1 tablespoon shredded coconut

Stir the milk, oats, and chia seeds together in a mason jar or bowl. Cover and refrigerate overnight. In the morning, top with almonds and coconut and enjoy.

NUTRITIONAL INFORMATION
One serving: Calories 397; Fat 11.5g (Sat 3.1g); Protein 15.6g; Carb 57.3g; Fiber 10.6g; Calcium 304mg; Iron 4.2mg; Sodium 96mg; Folate 45µg

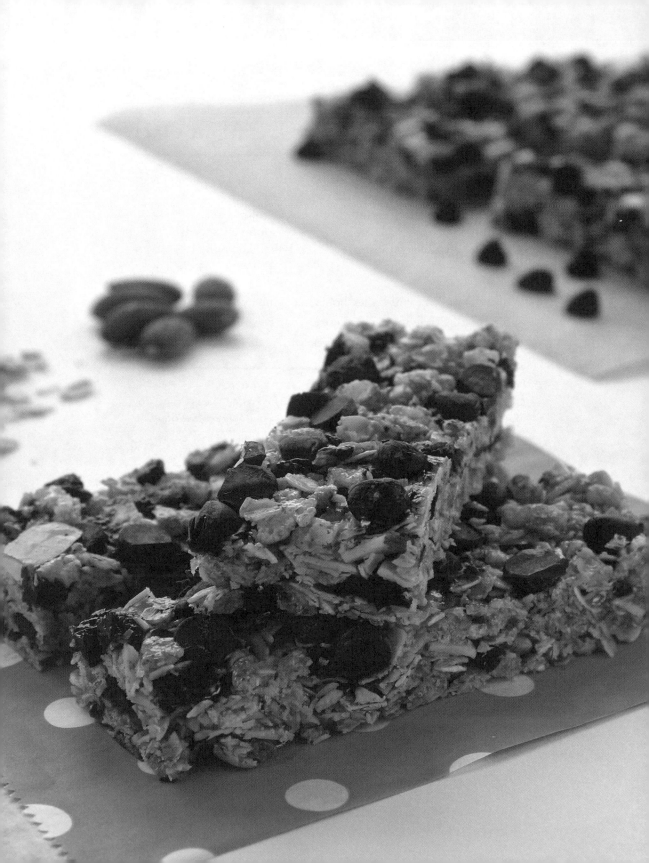

APPETIZERS, SNACKS, AND SANDWICHES

Roasted Sweet Potato Coins with Chipotle Crema

MAKES 8 SERVINGS

Your guests will rave about these adorable bites! Sweet potatoes contain an impressive array of nutrients including Vitamin A, Vitamin C, Vitamin B$_6$, manganese, potassium, and fiber. Slice them into "coins" and roast them in the oven for a delicious and healthy appetizer. I like to top mine with melted cheese and a chipotle crema, which supply plenty of calcium and protein.

Sweet Potato Coins
- 1½ pounds sweet potatoes (choose long, narrow potatoes)
- 1½ tablespoons olive oil
- ¾ teaspoon ground cumin
- ¾ teaspoon smoked paprika
- ½ teaspoon salt
- 1 cup shredded cheddar or Mexican blend cheese

Chipotle Crema
- ½ cup reduced-fat Greek yogurt or sour cream
- 1 teaspoon minced chipotles in adobo (more if you like it spicy)
- ½ teaspoon adobo sauce from the can
- 1 teaspoon lime juice
- ¼ cup sliced scallions

Preheat oven to 450°F. Wash the potatoes and slice them into ¼-inch slices or "coins." Place them in a bowl and add the oil, cumin, paprika, and salt. Toss to combine well. Arrange the potato coins on a baking sheet lined with parchment paper. Roast in the oven for 10 minutes, then flip and roast for another 10 minutes until tender. Remove the tray from the oven and sprinkle each coin with some cheese. Return the tray to the oven and cook for an additional 2 to 3 minutes until cheese is melted.

Meanwhile, make the chipotle crema by mixing the yogurt, chipotles, adobo sauce, and lime juice together in a small bowl.

Arrange the sweet potato coins on a serving platter. Top each with a dollop of chipotle crema. Garnish with scallions.

NUTRITIONAL INFORMATION
One serving: Calories 132; Fat 3.8g (Sat 1.1g); Protein 5.7g; Carb 19g; Fiber 2.8g; Calcium 116mg; Iron 0.8mg; Sodium 297mg; Folate 14µg

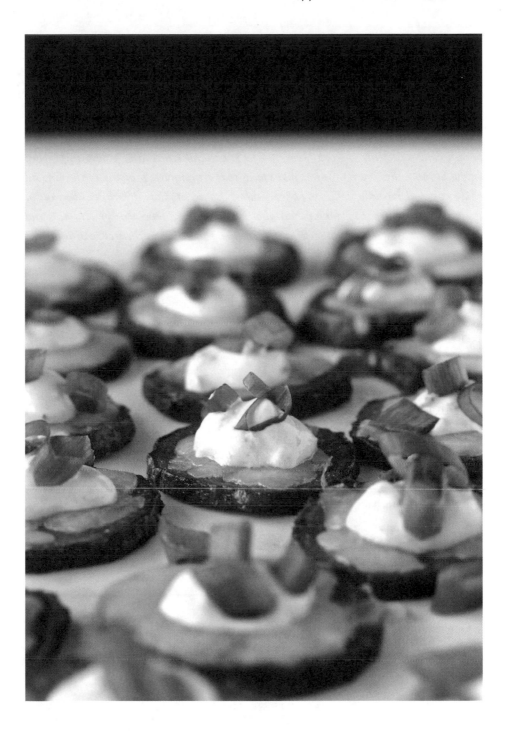

Wok-Charred Edamame with Sweet Soy Glaze

MAKES 4 SERVINGS

Edamame are the perfect pregnancy food. These young soybeans are low in calories and packed with nutrients so scoop them up by the handful (instead of potato chips) and enjoy! Soybeans are among the few plant foods that are complete proteins, containing all of the essential amino acids. They're also a fantastic source of folate, which is important in preventing birth defects. Edamame are also rich in fiber and several other vitamins and minerals including iron, calcium, zinc, and choline. Find them in the frozen aisle of your grocery store, shelled or in the pod.

1 bag (10 ounces) frozen edamame, in shell
1 tablespoon light soy sauce
1 tablespoon honey
½ teaspoon grated ginger
¼ teaspoon grated garlic
⅛ teaspoon red pepper flakes (optional)
1 tablespoon safflower, peanut, or other neutral-flavored oil

Cook the edamame according to package directions. Drain and set aside.

Mix the soy sauce, honey, ginger, garlic, and red pepper flakes together in a bowl.

Heat the oil in a wok over high heat. When the oil is very hot, add the edamame pods. Cook, stirring often, until the edamame becomes lightly charred, about 4 to 6 minutes.

Lower the heat to medium and let the wok cool down for a minute. Add the soy sauce mixture and toss to combine with the edamame. Cook, stirring constantly, until the sauce thickens and coats the edamame, about 30 seconds. Remove the edamame and serve.

NUTRITIONAL INFORMATION

One serving: Calories 125; Fat 3.3g (Sat 0.3g); Protein 7.5g; Carb 10.9g; Fiber 3.5g; Calcium 43mg; Iron 1.6mg; Sodium 137mg; Folate 215µg

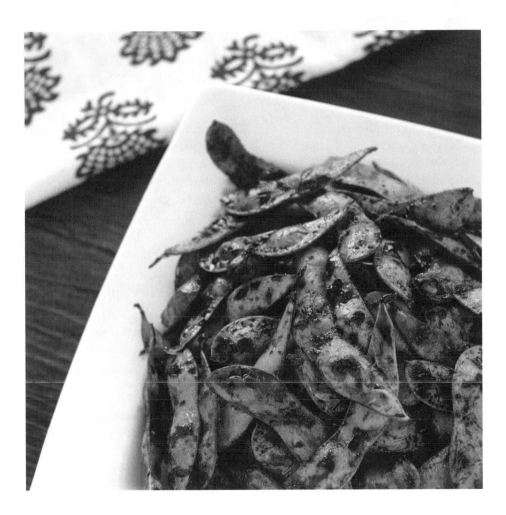

Spanish Garlic Shrimp (Gambas al Ajillo)

MAKES 6 APPETIZER SERVINGS OR 4 MAIN COURSE SERVINGS

In Spain, people enjoy tapas, which are small plates of food, to snack on with drinks before dinner. This sautéed shrimp dish is one of the most common tapas in Spain and it's also one of my favorites. It uses just a few simple ingredients but it's packed with flavor and beneficial nutrients. Olive oil provides heart-healthy monounsaturated fats and shrimp add protein, iron, Vitamin B$_{12}$, and brain-boosting omega-3 fatty acids. Be sure to serve this dish with Pan con Tomate (page 106) or other crusty bread to soak up the garlicky sauce.

4 tablespoons olive oil
4 cloves garlic, finely chopped
¼–½ teaspoon chili flakes
1 pound medium shrimp
1 teaspoon sweet Spanish paprika

¼ teaspoon salt
⅛ teaspoon pepper
2 tablespoons fresh lemon juice
3 tablespoons chopped parsley plus
  extra for garnish

Pour the oil into a large sauté pan and add garlic and chili flakes. Turn the heat up to medium high. As the pan heats up, the oil will slowly get infused with the flavor of the garlic and chili (do not let the garlic brown). Once the oil is hot and the garlic is fragrant, add the shrimp to the pan. Season them with the paprika, salt, and pepper. Cook the shrimp for 3 to 4 minutes, until they just turn pink, stirring them often. Add the lemon juice and parsley and cook for another minute or two until done (do not overcook the shrimp or they will turn rubbery).

Garnish with parsley and serve hot. Serve with Pan con Tomate (see page 106) for dipping.

NUTRITIONAL INFORMATION

One serving: Calories 191; Fat 11.5g (Sat 1.9g); Protein 12.6g; Carb 11.5g; Fiber 4.8g; Calcium 72mg; Iron 1.8mg; Sodium 434mg; Folate 36µg

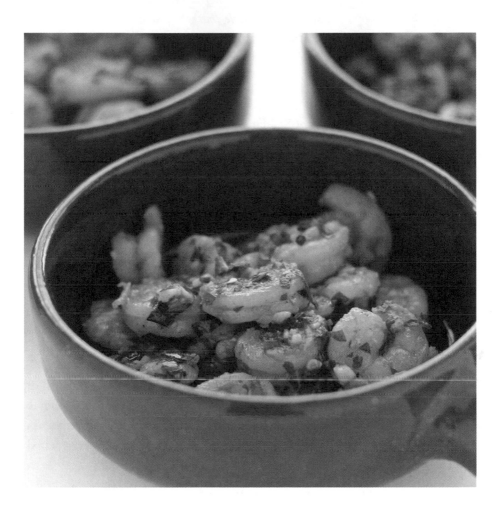

Cauliflower Cheesy Bread

attempted *didn't really* *"stick"*

MAKES 16 BREADSTICKS

Cauliflower forms the base of this healthy, gluten-free bread that's topped with cheesy goodness. Cauliflower is a cruciferous vegetable that's packed with powerful antioxidants as well as an impressive array of nutrients including protein, fiber, Vitamin C, Vitamin K, folate, and choline. Cheese adds a boost of calcium to the dish.

1 head cauliflower (about 2 pounds)
1 egg or 2 egg whites
1 cup shredded reduced-fat Cheddar Jack or other cheese, divided
1 teaspoon dried Italian seasoning

¼ teaspoons salt
⅛ teaspoon pepper
Marinara sauce for serving (optional)

Preheat oven to 450°F. Remove the outer leaves from the cauliflower and cut it into florets. Place the florets in the bowl of a food processor and pulse until it finely chopped (it should look like rice).

Transfer the cauliflower to a microwave-safe dish or bowl. Cover and cook in the microwave for 10 minutes. Alternatively, you can steam the cauliflower in a steamer basket or bake it in the oven at 375°F for 20 minutes.

When the cauliflower is cool, transfer it to a bowl lined with a kitchen towel or cheesecloth. Bring the ends of the cloth together and squeeze as much liquid out of the cauliflower as you can. Transfer the cauliflower to a mixing bowl and add the eggs, ½ cup cheese, Italian seasoning, salt, and pepper. Mix to combine.

Transfer the mixture to a baking sheet lined with parchment paper. Form the dough into a rectangle about 8 x 12 inches and ¼-inch thick. Bake in the oven for 15 to 20 minutes until cooked. Remove the baking sheet and sprinkle the remaining ½ cup cheese over the top. Bake for another 5 minutes until cheese is melted.

Cut into 16 breadsticks. Serve with marinara sauce for dipping.

NUTRITIONAL INFORMATION
One breadstick: Calories 26; Fat 0.8g (Sat 0.4g); Protein 2.8g; Carb 2g; Fiber 0.8g; Calcium 41mg; Iron 0.3mg; Sodium 58mg; Folate 23 µg

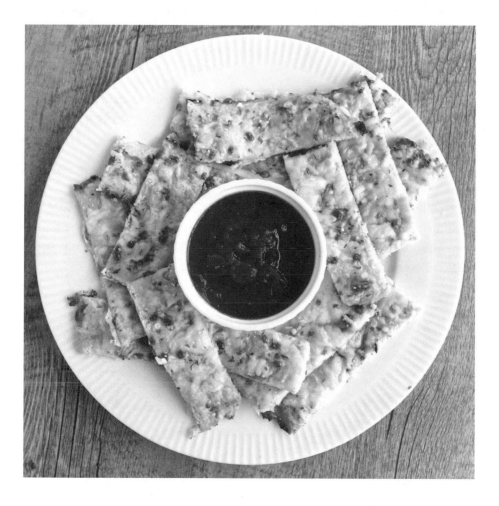

Pan con Tomate (Tomato Bread)

MAKES 8 SERVINGS

Sometimes the simplest dishes are the best. Originating in Catalonia, this tomato bread is one of the most common and well-loved dishes in Spain. A fresh loaf of bread is toasted and rubbed with garlic and tomato to give it a light coating of tomato pulp. It's finished with a drizzle of olive oil and a sprinkling of sea salt. Serve with Spanish Garlic Shrimp (page 102). This tasty dish provides heart-healthy monounsaturated fats and folate.

1 loaf ciabatta bread or baguette (about 12 ounces)
2 cloves garlic, peeled

2 medium, ripe Roma tomatoes
2 tablespoons extra virgin olive oil
Sea salt, to taste

Slice the loaf of bread in half horizontally. Toast the bread in a toaster oven or under a broiler until golden brown.

While the bread is still hot, rub the garlic all over the cut sides of the bread. Cut the tomatoes in half and rub the tomato on the bread, coating it with the tomato pulp. Drizzle the olive oil on top and sprinkle with sea salt. Serve immediately while still warm.

NUTRITIONAL INFORMATION
One serving: Calories 151; Fat 4.6g (Sat 0.8g); Protein 4.1g; Carb 22.7g; Fiber 1.5g; Calcium 37mg; Iron 1.4mg; Sodium 249mg; Folate 133µg

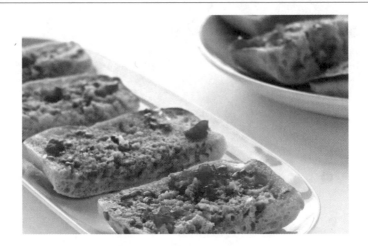

Greek Chicken Meatballs

MAKES 24 MEATBALLS OR 8 SERVINGS

These nutritious chicken meatballs are full of Greek flavor and are easy to make. Feta cheese and spinach help keep the meatballs moist. Spinach is a super food that's packed with a wide range of important pregnancy nutrients including fiber, protein, folate, calcium, and iron. These versatile meatballs freeze well so keep a batch ready for busy nights and add them to pasta dishes, soups, and sandwiches.

1 package (10 ounces) chopped, frozen spinach

1½ pounds ground chicken breast

3 cloves garlic, grated or minced

1 extra large egg

1 teaspoon dried oregano

1 teaspoon kosher salt

½ teaspoon black pepper

6 tablespoons crumbled pasteurized feta cheese

1 cup (2 ounces) fresh bread crumbs made from whole wheat bread (or ½ cup dried bread crumbs)

1 teaspoon olive oil

Preheat the oven to 400°F. Defrost the spinach according to package directions. Squeeze all of the water out of the spinach and place the spinach in a large bowl. Add all of the remaining ingredients except olive oil and mix gently to combine. Form the mixture into 24 meatballs, about 1½ inches in diameter.

Grease a baking sheet with the olive oil. Place the meatballs on the baking sheet and bake in the oven, about 15 to 18 minutes, until lightly golden and cooked through. Serve warm.

NUTRITIONAL INFORMATION
One serving (3 meatballs): Calories 160; Fat 4.3g (Sat 1.9g); Protein 22.2g; Carb 5.4g; Fiber 1.7g; Calcium 102mg; Iron 1.5mg; Sodium 537mg; Folate 64µg

To make fresh bread crumbs, break 2 slices of bread into pieces and pulse in a mini food processor until crumbs form. To make this recipe gluten free, substitute ½ ground oats (certified gluten free).

Sesame Noodles with Broccoli

MAKES 4 SERVINGS

Peanut butter, sesame oil, and soy sauce come together with ginger and garlic in this addictive noodle dish that requires minimal cooking time. It makes a perfect appetizer or picnic dish and can be served hot, cold, or at room temperature. Add some grilled chicken or tofu and it becomes a substantial main course. This dish is packed with protein and folate and also provides a good amount of fiber and iron. Broccoli is also rich in Vitamin C, which helps your body absorb the iron in the dish.

8 ounces whole grain spaghetti

1 tablespoon sesame oil

2 teaspoons safflower, peanut, or other neutral-flavored oil

1 teaspoon grated or finely chopped ginger

1 teaspoon grated or finely chopped garlic

½–1 teaspoon Asian chile paste such as Sambal Oelek

5 tablespoons creamy natural peanut butter

1½ tablespoons reduced-sodium soy sauce

2 teaspoons rice vinegar

2 teaspoons packed brown sugar

⅓ cup water

4 cups steamed broccoli florets

1 teaspoon toasted sesame seeds for garnish

2 scallions, thinly sliced on a diagonal for garnish

Bring a large pot of water to a boil. Add the spaghetti and cook according to package directions. Drain and rinse with cold water. Toss with sesame oil to prevent the noodles from sticking. Set aside.

While the spaghetti is cooking, heat the oil in a medium saucepan over medium heat. Add the ginger, garlic, and chili paste and cook until fragrant, about 30 seconds. Add the peanut butter, soy sauce, vinegar, sugar, and water and stir to combine. Cook for 3 to 4 minutes until the sugar has dissolved and the sauce is smooth.

Pour the sauce over the spaghetti. Add the broccoli and toss to combine. Garnish with sesame seeds and scallions. Can be served hot, cold, or at room temperature.

NUTRITIONAL INFORMATION

One serving: Calories 414; Fat 16.1g (Sat 3g); Protein 15.2g; Carb 53g; Fiber 3.4g; Calcium 70mg; Iron 3.2mg; Sodium 227mg; Folate 292µg

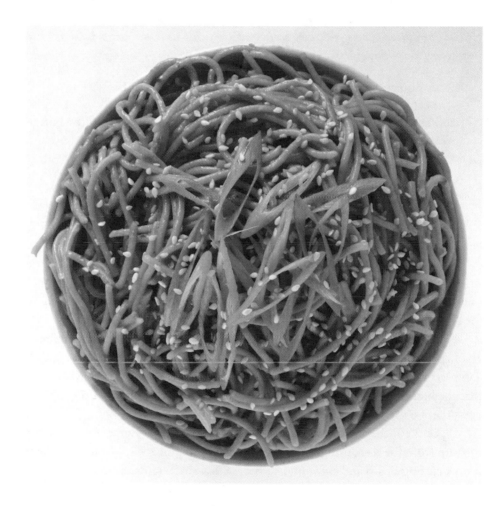

No-Bake Chocolate Cherry Granola Bars

MAKES 12 BARS

These healthy no-bake granola bars are the ideal portable breakfast or snack. The combination of heart-healthy oats along with rice cereal gives them the perfect chewy yet crispy texture. Almonds and flaxseed along with dried cherries and dark chocolate add flavor as well as fiber, protein, omega–3 fatty acids, and antioxidants. Once you make a batch of these, you'll never buy granola bars again.

1½ cups quick-cooking oats
 (not rolled oats)
1 cup enriched puffed rice cereal
 (like Rice Krispies®)
¼ cup sliced almonds
¼ cup ground flaxseed or
 wheat germ

¼ cup packed light brown sugar
¼ cup honey
¼ cup coconut oil or unsalted butter
1 teaspoon vanilla extract
¼ teaspoon salt
½ cup dried cherries, chopped
⅓ cup dark chocolate chips

Line an 8 x 8-inch square baking dish with parchment paper or aluminum foil, letting the ends hang over the sides of the dish.

Mix the oats, rice cereal, almonds, and flaxseed together in a bowl. Heat the sugar, honey, and coconut oil in a large saucepan on the stove, stirring often until the sugar dissolves. Bring to a boil, and then lower to a simmer. Simmer the mixture for 2 minutes. Remove the pan from the heat and stir in the vanilla and salt.

Pour the oat mixture into the saucepan. Using a spatula, stir well to combine all of the ingredients. Stir in the cherries. Transfer the mixture to the baking dish and press it down into the pan, packing it in firmly (packing it in tightly will ensure that the bars don't fall apart). Sprinkle the chocolate chips evenly over the top and press them lightly into the granola mixture.

Place the dish in the refrigerator and chill for 2 hours. Remove the granola mixture from the dish, using the parchment paper to pull it out of the dish. Place it on a cutting board and cut it into 12 bars with a sharp knife. Store extra bars in the refrigerator with parchment paper or foil in between the layers to prevent them from sticking.

NUTRITIONAL INFORMATION
One bar: Calories 197; Fat 9.3g (Sat 5.7g); Protein 3g; Carb 25.5g; Fiber 2.8g; Calcium 25mg; Iron 1.6mg; Sodium 52mg; Folate 7µg

Quick-cooking oats are the same as rolled or old-fashioned oats but they are coarsely chopped so that they cook faster. If you only have rolled oats, you can give them a quick whir in the food processor to make quick-cooking oats. Use about 1¾ cup rolled oats to yield 1½ cups quick oats.

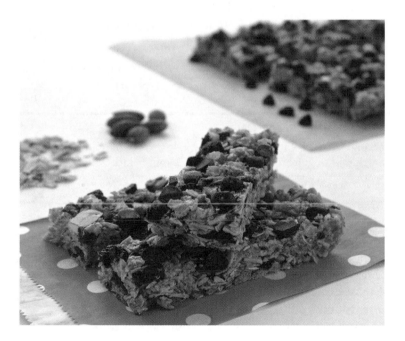

Avocado Toast

MAKES 2 SERVINGS

Avocado toast has become something of a culinary phenomenon recently. It's the ultimate healthy snack and it has an endless number of variations. Plus, it only takes 5 minutes to prepare—how can you beat that? With nearly 20 vitamins and minerals in every serving, avocados are nutritional rock stars! They also are a rich source of heart-healthy monounsaturated fats, fiber, and folate. Use whole grain toast as your base to increase the health benefits of this dish. Below is a classic recipe, along with two variations.

2 slices whole grain bread
1 medium ripe avocado

1 teaspoon fresh lemon juice
Olive oil and sea salt, for garnish

Toast the bread. Slice the avocado in half lengthwise and remove the pit. Scoop the flesh out with a spoon and place it in a bowl. Add the lemon juice and coarsely mash the avocado with a fork.

Spread the avocado on the toast, drizzle with olive oil and sprinkle sea salt on top. Cut each piece in half and serve.

NUTRITIONAL INFORMATION
One serving: Calories 230; Fat 14.6g (Sat 2.4g); Protein 5.6g; Carb 20.3g; Fiber 8.7g; Calcium 41mg; Iron 1.2mg; Sodium 139mg; Folate 95µg

Chili Lime Avocado Toast

⅛ teaspoon chili flakes
½ teaspoon ground cumin
1 teaspoon lime juice (replacing lemon juice above)
Toasted pepitas, for garnish

Mash the avocado with ⅛ teaspoon chili flakes, ½ teaspoon ground cumin, and 1 teaspoon lime juice (instead of lemon juice). Spread avocado on toast and top with toasted pepitas (pumpkin seeds), olive oil, and sea salt.

Feta and Radish Avocado Toast

3 tablespoons feta cheese, crumbled
Sliced radishes, for garnish

Coarsely mash the avocado with lemon juice and 3 tablespoons crumbled feta cheese. Spread avocado on toast and top with sliced radishes, olive oil, and sea salt.

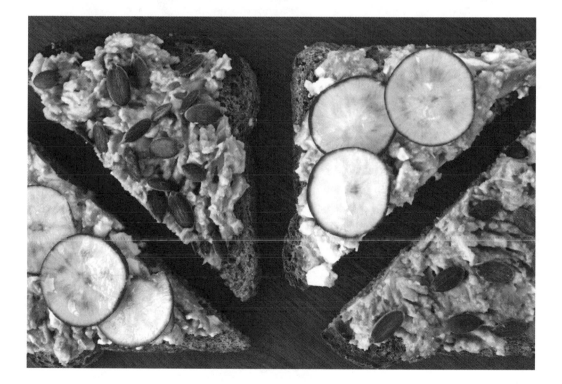

Simply Delicious Hummus

MAKES 1½ CUPS OR 6 SERVINGS

It's so easy to make hummus at home—once you try it, you'll probably never buy it again. My hummus uses the classic combination of chickpeas and tahini paste, but adds sesame oil to the mix to enhance the flavors. Tahini paste, which is made from ground sesame seeds, can be found in specialty grocery stores. Hummus is a great vegetarian source of protein and fiber, as well as several other nutrients like folate, iron, and calcium. Use it as a dip for vegetables and pretzels, or as a spread on sandwiches instead of mayonnaise. This is a good base recipe to which you can add your favorite ingredients. Try jarred roasted red peppers for a smoky version or chipotles in adobo, if you like spice.

1 can (15 ounces) reduced-sodium chickpeas, rinsed and drained
1 small clove (or ½ regular clove) garlic
2 tablespoons tahini paste
2 tablespoons fresh lemon juice
¼ teaspoon ground cumin
1 tablespoon olive oil plus extra for drizzling on top
1½ teaspoons sesame oil
3 tablespoons water
1 teaspoon za'atar (can substitute ½ teaspoon smoked paprika)
Salt and pepper, to taste

Place the chickpeas, garlic, tahini paste, lemon juice, and cumin together in a food processor and pulse until finely chopped. With the motor still running, pour in the olive oil and sesame oil. Add the water and continue to blend until smooth. Season with salt and pepper to taste.

Transfer hummus to a serving bowl, drizzle with olive oil and sprinkle with za'atar or smoked paprika.

NUTRITIONAL INFORMATION
One serving: Calories 149; Fat 6.9g (Sat 1g); Protein 4.5g; Carb 17.9g; Fiber 3.5g; Calcium 32mg; Iron 1.3mg; Sodium 213mg; Folate 53µg

---

Za'atar is a Middle Eastern dried spice mix with sumac, sesame seeds, and other spices like oregano and thyme.

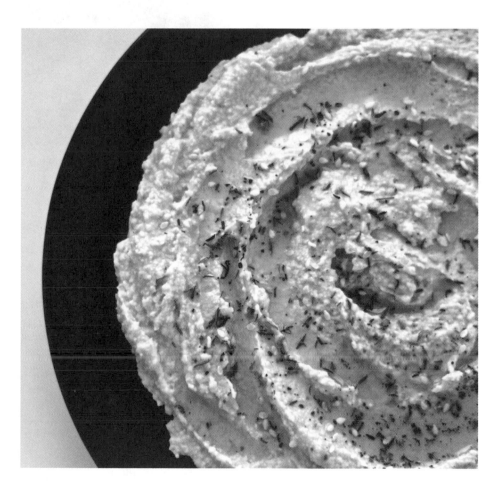

Crispy Spiced Chickpeas

MAKES 4 SERVINGS (2 CUPS)

These tasty morsels are dusted with Moroccan spices and roasted in the oven until crispy. My Crispy Spiced Chickpeas are the perfect snack—healthy, satisfying and portable. Keep them in a plastic bag and take them on the go so you have something to reach for when hunger strikes. Chickpeas are a terrific vegetarian source of protein and fiber. They also provide several important nutrients, including folate, iron, and calcium. Feel free to mix up the spices to create your own perfect blend.

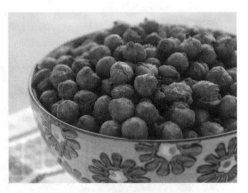

2 cans (15.5 ounce each) low-sodium chickpeas, drained and rinsed
2 tablespoons olive oil
2 teaspoons smoked paprika
1 teaspoon cumin
1 teaspoon coriander
¼ teaspoon cayenne pepper
¼ teaspoon salt

Preheat oven to 400° F. Dry the chickpeas with a kitchen towel and place them in a bowl. Add the oil and spices and toss to combine well.

Spread the chickpeas out in a single layer on a baking sheet. Roast in the oven, stirring once or twice, until chickpeas are dry and crispy, about 35 to 40 minutes.

Let the chickpeas cool before serving (they will crisp up more as they dry). Store in an airtight container.

NUTRITIONAL INFORMATION
One serving: Calories 268; Fat 10.3g (Sat 1g); Protein 10.5g; Carb 35g; Fiber 9.1g; Calcium 80mg; Iron 3.7mg; Sodium 383mg; Folate 147µg

Refrigerator Dill Pickles

MAKES ABOUT 5 SERVINGS

Crunchy, refreshing and delightfully tangy—who doesn't love a good pickle? One of the most common pregnancy cravings, dill pickles are actually a cinch to make at home. A simple brine gets poured over cucumbers and transforms them into pickles. Although you can eat them right away, they're even better after they've had time to soak overnight. Cucumbers provide a good amount of Vitamin C, Vitamin K and potassium, and are also packed with water to help keep you hydrated.

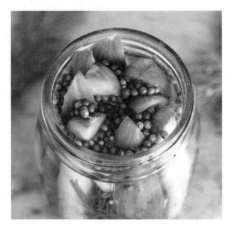

¾ cup distilled white vinegar
1¼ cups water
2 tablespoons kosher salt
1 tablespoon plus 1 teaspoon sugar
4 cloves garlic, peeled
⅛ teaspoon red pepper flakes
12 sprigs fresh dill

1 tablespoon coriander seeds (optional)
1 teaspoon mustard seeds (optional)
1 pound mini cucumbers or Kirby cucumbers (about 5 mini pickles), cut into spears

Heat the vinegar, water, salt, and sugar together in a medium saucepan, stirring occasionally, until the salt and sugar are dissolved. Remove from heat and cool.

Divide the garlic, chili flakes, dill, coriander seeds, and mustard seeds between two standard (1½ cup) mason jars. Place the cucumber spears in the jars, packing them in to fit. Pour the brine mixture into the jars. Add water as needed to cover the cucumbers with liquid. Close the jars and refrigerate for 24 hours before serving. Store the pickles in a sealed jar in the fridge.

NUTRITIONAL INFORMATION
One serving: Calories 41; Fat 0.4g (Sat 0.1g); Protein 1g; Carb 8.2g; Fiber 1g; Calcium 32mg; Iron 0.6mg; Folate 7µg

---

Deviled Egg Spread

MAKES 6 SERVINGS

This recipe was shared by my dear friend Ann from the Fountain Avenue Kitchen (www. fountainavenuekitchen.com). Besides being a talented cook, blogger and writer, she's also the mom of two handsome boys. What I love about this recipe is that it has all of the flavor of deviled eggs with none of the fuss! No need to stuff any eggs—simply mix the ingredients together, spread it on some whole grain toast, add any additional toppings and you're good to go. This dish packs a protein punch and also supplies plenty of choline, which is essential for the development of your baby's brain.

6 hard-boiled eggs
2 tablespoons reduced-fat Greek
    yogurt
2 tablespoons mayonnaise
1 teaspoon Dijon mustard
¼ teaspoon Worcestershire sauce
¼ teaspoon kosher or sea salt

⅛ teaspoon black pepper
Optional toppings or mix-ins:
    chopped greens olives, avocado,
    fresh basil, or dill
Toasted whole-grain bread (or bread
    of choice) or tomatoes for serving

Slice the eggs in half, remove the yolks, and place the yolks in a mixing bowl. Mash the yolks and then add the yogurt, mayonnaise, Dijon, Worcestershire, salt, and pepper.

Chop the egg whites and add them to the bowl along with any optional add-ins. Stir to combine. Spread the mixture on toast or scoop into a hollowed-out tomato. Scatter optional garnishes on top.

NUTRITIONAL INFORMATION
One serving: Calories 116; Fat 8.3g (Sat 2.2g); Protein 6.6g; Carb 1g; Fiber 0g; Calcium 34mg; Iron 0.6mg; Sodium 209mg; Folate 22mg

Crispy Kale Chips

MAKES 8 SERVINGS

The next time you're craving potato chips, try these crispy kale chips instead. These chips are light, nutritious and a cinch to make. Kale is truly a super food! It's packed with vitamins, especially Vitamins A, C, and K. It also supplies several important minerals including calcium, potassium, and iron. And if that wasn't enough, kale also contains powerful antioxidants, fiber, and protein. This recipe simply calls for salt but you can also sprinkle on your favorite spices before baking in the oven.

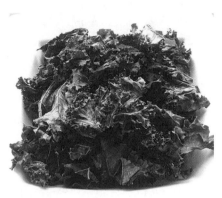

1 bunch curly or Tuscan kale
   (12 ounces)

1½ tablespoons olive oil
Kosher salt, to taste

Preheat oven to 325°F. Rinse and dry the kale leaves. Make sure the kale leaves are completely dry so that they crisp up nicely in the oven. Remove the stems and ribs, then cut or tear the leaves into large pieces. Toss the kale pieces in a large bowl with the olive oil and mix with your hands to make sure all of the pieces are coated. Season them with salt.

    Transfer the kale to two baking sheets, arranging the pieces in a single layer. Bake in the oven until crispy, about 10 minutes. Watch them carefully during the last few minutes as they can burn quickly. Remove the tray from the oven and let the chips cool before serving.

NUTRITIONAL INFORMATION
One serving: Calories 43; Fat 2.7g (Sat 0.4g); Protein 1.4g; Carb 4.3g; Fiber 0.9g; Calcium 57mg; Iron 0.7mg; Sodium 18mg; Folate 12mg

Tropical Popcorn Trail Mix

MAKES 6 SERVINGS

Skip the chips and candy and bring on the popcorn! Whole grains, fiber, and antioxidants are all wrapped up in this tasty snack. Popcorn is satisfying and affordable and it's a great addition to roasted nuts and dried fruit in this easy trail mix. And, did you know that it's a whole grain? Be careful though as many brands of microwave popcorn are packed with partially hydrogenated oils and sodium. The healthiest way to make popcorn is with an air popper so that you can add your own toppings. A good tip is to use an olive oil sprayer to lightly coat the kernels with oil—you'll end up using a lot less.

6 cups air popped popcorn
Olive oil (use an oil sprayer)
1 cup mixed nuts (like almonds, cashews, Brazil nuts, walnuts, and pecans)

1 cup mixed dried fruit (like banana chips, pineapple, mango, and apricots)
¼ cup dried unsweetened coconut flakes
Sea salt, to taste

Place the popcorn in a large bowl and spray the kernels with olive oil until lightly coated. Season with salt to taste. Add the nuts, fruit, and coconut flakes and toss to combine.

NUTRITIONAL INFORMATION
One serving: Calories 225; Fat 14.3g (Sat 3.6g); Protein 6.6g; Carb 19.6g; Fiber 5.4g; Calcium 68mg; Iron 1.5mg; Sodium 2mg; Folate 15mg

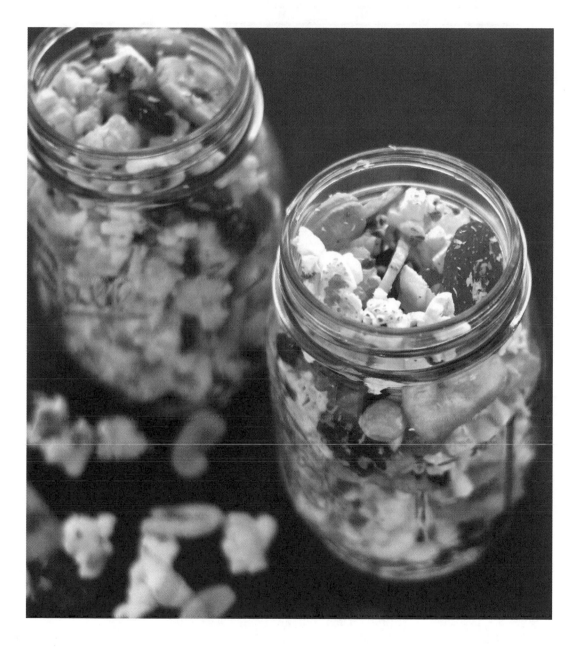

Snack Attack Spiced Nuts

MAKES 2½ CUPS OR 10 SERVINGS

A combination of nutrient-rich nuts are dipped in egg whites and coated in a mixture of spices with an irresistible combination of sweet, spicy, and smoky flavors. These spiced nuts are the perfect on-the-go snack and they also make great holiday gifts. Nuts are packed with heart-healthy fats, protein, fiber, and several vitamins and minerals that are beneficial for your health.

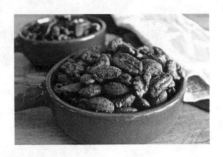

¼ cup packed light brown sugar
1 tablespoon cinnamon
1 teaspoon kosher salt
½ teaspoon cumin
¼–½ teaspoon cayenne pepper
   (depending on how spicy you
   like it)

1 egg white
2½ cups assorted nuts such as
   walnuts, almonds, and pecans

Preheat oven to 350°F. Mix the brown sugar, cinnamon, salt, cumin, and cayenne pepper together in a medium bowl. Whip the egg white in another bowl with a whisk until light and frothy. Drop the nuts into the bowl and toss to combine. Remove the nuts, shaking off any excess egg white, and drop them into the bowl with the spice mix. Toss to coat all of the nuts with the spices.

Spray a baking sheet with nonstick cooking spray or line the sheet with a nonstick baking mat. Spread the nuts on the sheet in a single layer and bake in the oven for 15 minutes, stirring once halfway through. Remove the nuts and let them cool on a wire rack. As they cool, they will crisp up. Serve right away or store in an airtight container for one week.

NUTRITIONAL INFORMATION
One serving: Calories 224; Fat 16.7g (Sat 1.2g); Protein 8g; Carb 11.6g; Fiber 3.7g; Calcium 70mg; Iron 1.3mg; Sodium 239mg; Folate 13mg

Quick Pickled Shallots

MAKES 1 CUP

An easy way to add acidity and crunch to a dish, these pickled shallots pack a flavor punch. Shallots are milder than regular onions and may be gentler on your stomach, but if you can't find them you can substitute red onions. Add them to sandwiches or serve them with Roasted Sweet Potato and Black Bean Tacos (see page 210).

½ cup red wine vinegar
½ cup water
1 tablespoon honey

1 teaspoon kosher salt
1 cup thinly sliced shallots
   (about 8 shallots)

Mix the vinegar, water, honey, and salt together in a bowl. Add the shallots and stir to combine. Cover and let sit at room temperature for 1 hour. Drain and serve.

NUTRITIONAL INFORMATION
One serving (2 tablespoons): Calories 25; Fat 0g (Sat 0g); Protein 0.5g; Carb 5.6g; Fiber 0g; Calcium 8mg; Iron 0.3mg; Folate 6mg

Homemade Vegan Mayonnaise

MAKES 1 CUP

You won't go back to store-bought mayonnaise after trying this dish. My vegan mayonnaise is lower in calories and fat than traditional mayo. Believe it or not, it's made with tofu, which provides protein, calcium, and iron. Simply throw all of the ingredients together in a blender and the result is a healthy spread with a texture and flavor that's surprisingly close to classic mayonnaise. Tofu makes a great canvas for other flavors, so feel free to experiment with different varieties. Add some fresh basil for an Italian version or chipotles in adobo and lime juice for a Mexican spin.

8 ounces firm tofu, drained
2 teaspoons Dijon mustard
1 tablespoon cider vinegar
2 teaspoons fresh lemon juice

¼ teaspoon salt
3 tablespoons safflower, grapeseed,
   or other neutral-flavored oil

Place all ingredients in a blender and blend until smooth. Store mayonnaise in an airtight container in the refrigerator.

NUTRITIONAL INFORMATION
One serving (2 tablespoons): Calories 68; Fat 6.1g (Sat 0.6g); Protein 2.3g; Carb 0.6g; Fiber 0.3g; Calcium 57mg; Iron 0.5mg; Sodium 107mg; Folate 5mg

Roasted Vegetable Hummus Wraps

MAKES 6 SERVINGS

These meatless wraps are packed with complex carbohydrates, protein, and fiber to satisfy your appetite and keep you energized. They're also rich in several vitamins and minerals including folate.

1½ cups Simply Delicious Hummus (see page 114) or store-bought hummus
6 whole wheat wraps

Oven-Roasted Vegetables (see page 224)
2 cups baby spinach leaves

To assemble the wraps, spread 2 tablespoons hummus down the center of each wrap. Top with equal amounts of roasted vegetables and spinach. Fold the ends of the wraps in and roll them up like a burrito. Cut in half on a diagonal and serve.

NUTRITIONAL INFORMATION
One serving: Calories 379; Fat 13.6g (Sat 1.7g); Protein 11g; Carb 56.9g; Fiber 9.9g; Calcium 83mg; Iron 2.3mg; Sodium 586mg; Folate 118µg

Brain-Boosting Salmon Burgers

MAKES 6 BURGERS

These burgers are a great way to incorporate nutritious seafood into your diet. After all, who doesn't love burgers? The patties can be frozen and heated up for a quick weeknight meal. Salmon is one of the richest sources of omega-3 fatty acids and it's packed with an abundance of vitamins, minerals, and protein. This recipe is also a good source of calcium, iron, and folate.

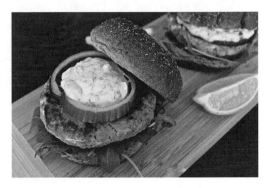

Burgers

1½ pounds skinless salmon fillet, preferably wild Alaskan
3 scallions, sliced
1 tablespoon Dijon mustard
1 tablespoon reduced-fat mayonnaise
1½ teaspoon Old Bay seasoning
2 teaspoons lemon juice plus 1

teaspoon lemon zest
1 ounce fresh whole wheat bread crumbs (about ½ cup) made from 1 slice of bread
1 teaspoon hot sauce like Sriracha
½ teaspoon kosher salt
¼ teaspoon black pepper

Dill Yogurt Sauce

¾ cup reduced-fat or nonfat Greek yogurt
1½ tablespoons fresh, chopped dill
2 teaspoons lemon juice
Salt and pepper, to taste

Olive oil cooking spray
6 multigrain hamburger rolls, toasted
Assorted toppings, like baby arugula or spinach and red onion slices

Finely dice half of the salmon into pieces about ¼-inch in size. Cut the remainder of the salmon roughly into chunks and place them in a food processor. Pulse until a paste forms. Transfer the paste to a large bowl and add the diced salmon, scallions, mustard, mayonnaise, Old Bay, lemon juice, zest, bread crumbs, hot sauce, salt, and pepper. Gently mix the ingredients together until combined. Form the mixture into 6 equal patties.

To make the sauce, mix the yogurt, dill, and lemon juice together in a small bowl. Season with salt and pepper.

Spray a large nonstick skillet with olive oil spray and heat over medium high heat. Add the burgers (working in batches if needed) and cook for 3 to 4 minutes, until browned on the bottom. Flip the burgers over and cook for an additional 3 to 4 minutes until cooked through. Serve the burgers on toasted buns with dill yogurt sauce and desired toppings.

NUTRITIONAL INFORMATION
One serving: Calories 372; Fat 12.5g (Sat 3.2g); Protein 29.5g; Carb 24.5g; Fiber 2.2g; Calcium 155mg; Iron 2.9mg; Sodium 745mg; Folate 84mg

To make the fresh bread crumbs, remove the crusts from a slice of whole wheat bread and tear the bread into pieces. Pulse in a food processor until crumbs form. Can substitute ¼ cup dried whole wheat bread crumbs.

Black Bean and Quinoa Veggie Burgers

MAKES 8 BURGERS

If you're not a fan of veggie burgers, hopefully this recipe will change your mind. It's actually the all-time most popular recipe on my blog (www.thefoodiephysician.com). These burgers have it all! Black beans, quinoa, and oats provide plenty of complex carbohydrates, protein, and fiber to give you long-lasting energy and keep you satisfied. They're also rich in

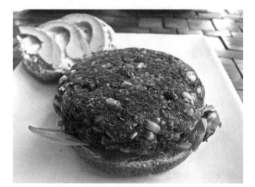

calcium, iron, and folate. These burgers freeze well, so pack them away—they'll come in handy after baby arrives.

Patties

½ cup quinoa
1 teaspoon olive oil
1 small red onion, chopped
3 cloves garlic, minced
2 cans low-sodium black beans (15.5 ounces each), rinsed and drained
2 tablespoons tomato paste
1 large egg

⅔ cup cooked corn (canned or fresh)
¼ cup chopped cilantro
1 tablespoon minced chipotles in adobo
1½ teaspoons ground cumin
½ teaspoon kosher salt
1 cup rolled oats, ground into crumbs

Yogurt Sauce

½ cup reduced-fat or nonfat Greek yogurt
1 teaspoon minced chipotles in adobo + ½ teaspoon adobo sauce from the can
1 teaspoon honey

½ teaspoon Dijon mustard
6 whole wheat hamburger rolls, lightly toasted
Lettuce, avocado slices, and tomatoes for toppings (optional)

Place the quinoa in a small saucepan along with 1 cup of water. Bring the water to a boil, and then reduce heat to medium low and cover the pan. Cook for 10 to 15 minutes until the water is absorbed and quinoa is cooked. Remove from heat.

Heat the oil in a small sauté pan over medium heat and add the onion and garlic. Sauté until onions are softened, about 5 to 6 minutes. Place the mixture into a large bowl. Add approximately 1½ cans of black beans to the bowl. Using a potato masher or fork, mash all of the ingredients together until a pasty mixture forms.

Stir in the remaining beans, along with the tomato paste, egg, corn, cilantro, chipotles, cumin, and salt. Stir in the cooked quinoa and ground oats until evenly distributed.

Form the mixture into eight equal patties, compacting them well with your hands as you form them. Place the patties on a baking sheet, cover them with plastic wrap, and refrigerate for at least a few hours or overnight.

To make the yogurt sauce, stir the yogurt, chipotles, adobo sauce, honey, and mustard together in a small bowl.

When ready to eat, preheat the oven to 400°F. Spray a baking sheet with non-stick cooking spray and place the patties on the sheet. Cook for 10 to 12 minutes until the patties are golden brown and crispy, then carefully flip them over and cook another 10 minutes. Serve patties on the buns with the yogurt sauce and toppings of your choice.

NUTRITIONAL INFORMATION
One serving: Calories 414; Fat 6.6g (Sat 1.4g); Protein 18g; Carb 72.2g; Fiber 10.9g; Calcium 97mg; Iron 4mg; Sodium 596mg; Folate 113mg

---

Chipotle Burgers with Avocado Crema

MAKES 4 BURGERS

These tasty burgers are leaner than traditional burgers and packed with nutrients. Mixing onions and spices into the patties keeps them moist and flavorful. The burgers are topped with a cooling crema made with nutritious avocado. Beef is rich in protein, iron, Vitamin B$_{12}$, and zinc. This dish also supplies a good amount of fiber, calcium, and folate.

Patties
1 pound 93% lean ground beef
3 tablespoons grated onion
1 clove garlic, grated or minced
1 teaspoon minced chipotle in adobo
 (plus 2 teaspoons adobo sauce)

¾ teaspoon salt
¼ teaspoon black pepper`

Avocado crema
1 medium avocado (preferably Haas
 avocado)
2 tablespoons nonfat Greek yogurt

2 teaspoons lime juice
1 tablespoon chopped cilantro
Salt, to taste

Oil for brushing the grill rack
2 ounces reduced-fat cheddar
 cheese, shredded

4 whole wheat hamburger buns
1 tomato, sliced

Preheat grill to medium high heat. Mix the beef, onion, garlic, chipotles, adobo sauce, salt, and pepper together. Be careful not to overwork the meat. Form into patties, making an indentation in the center of each burger so that they will cook evenly.

Mix all of the avocado crema ingredients together in a bowl. Set aside.

Brush the grill rack with oil. Place the burger patties on the rack and cook for 4 to 5 minutes on each side for medium. Place the cheese on the patties during the last 2 minutes of grilling. Place the buns, cut side down, on the outer edges of the rack to toast lightly during the last minute of grilling.

To assemble the burgers, place a cheese-topped patty on each bun bottom and top with a slice of tomato and ¼ of the avocado crema. Add bun tops and serve.

NUTRITIONAL INFORMATION
One serving: Calories 381; Fat 16.1g (Sat 5g); Protein 32.4g; Carb 25.6g; Fiber 4.6g; Calcium 140mg; Iron 4.6mg; Sodium 810mg; Folate 129µg

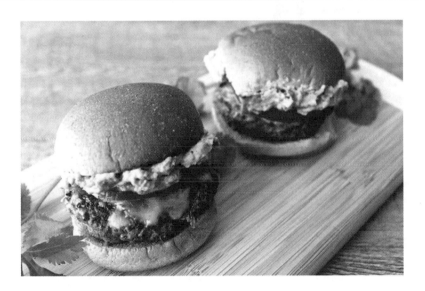

Turkey Parmesan Burgers

MAKES 4 BURGERS

These turkey burgers are sure to be a hit with your family. They're bursting with Italian flavors and stay moist thanks to the addition of marinara sauce in the patties. They're packed with protein, fiber, and zinc and also supply a good amount of iron and calcium.

1 pound lean ground turkey (or chicken)
6 tablespoons marinara sauce, divided use
1 clove garlic, minced
2 tablespoons grated Parmesan cheese
½ teaspoon dried oregano
¼ teaspoon dried thyme
¼ teaspoon kosher salt

⅛ teaspoon black pepper
¼ teaspoon red pepper flakes
2 teaspoons olive oil
½ cup shredded part-skim mozzarella cheese
4 whole grain hamburger buns or 8 slices whole grain bread, toasted
Handful of fresh basil leaves or arugula

Mix the turkey, 2 tablespoons marinara sauce, garlic, cheese, oregano, thyme, salt, pepper, and red pepper flakes together in a large bowl. Form into four patties.

Heat the oil in a large nonstick skillet over medium high heat and add the patties. Cook for 4 to 5 minutes, then flip and cook for another 4 to 5 minutes until completely cooked through. During the last minute of cooking, add 2 tablespoons shredded cheese on top of each burger and cover the skillet to melt the cheese.

To serve, place the patties on toasted hamburger buns or bread. Top each patty with 1 tablespoon marinara sauce and a few basil or arugula leaves. Add the bun tops and serve.

NUTRITIONAL INFORMATION
One serving: Calories 397; Fat 15.8g (Sat 5.2g); Protein 33.5g; Carb 27.6g; Fiber 4.7g; Calcium 235mg; Iron 3.2mg; Sodium 711mg; Folate 41mg

Green Grilled Cheese Sandwich

MAKES 2 SERVINGS

This genius recipe is from Justine, one half of the team over at Full Belly Sisters (www. fullbellysisters.blogspot.com). She takes the traditional grilled cheese to a new level and adds a boost of nutrition with the addition of avocado and spinach. Both are rich sources of folate, a crucial pregnancy nutrient. This dish also provides plenty of protein, calcium, and fiber.

1½ cups baby spinach
¼ medium avocado
3 ounces smoked Gouda or extra
   sharp cheddar, roughly chopped
2 slices peasant bread

2 teaspoons extra virgin olive oil
Salt, to taste
Tabasco or other hot sauce
   (optional)

Pack the spinach into a small food processor and chop. Add the avocado and process a bit more until it turns into a paste. Add the cheese and pulse a few more times until the pieces are small and dispersed throughout. If you'd prefer to shred it, just fold the shredded cheese into the avocado-spinach paste. Taste and season with salt and hot sauce.

Spread the mixture evenly over the slices of bread and close them to form a sandwich. Brush some oil on the outside, and grill the sandwich for a couple of minutes on each side in a pan over medium-high heat. The bread should be golden and crispy and the cheese should be ooey-gooey. Cut in half and serve. Keep a napkin handy!

Note: you can also serve this as two open-faced sandwiches. Place them under the broiler until the cheese melts.

NUTRITIONAL INFORMATION
One serving: Calories 316; Fat 19.8g (Sat 8.9g); Protein 14.4g; Carb 18.9g; Fiber 3g; Calcium 345mg; Iron 1.8mg; Sodium 542mg; Folate 163mg

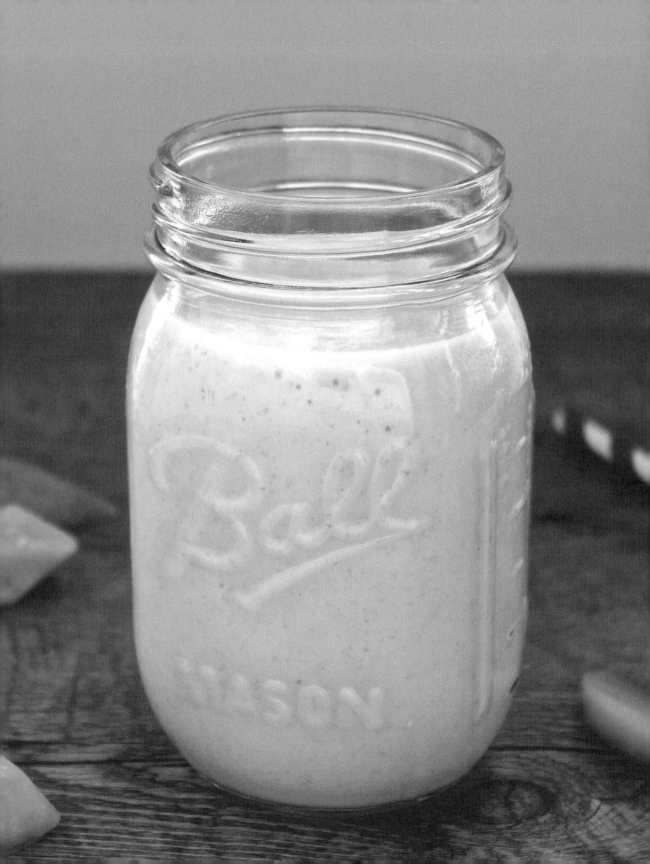

BEVERAGES

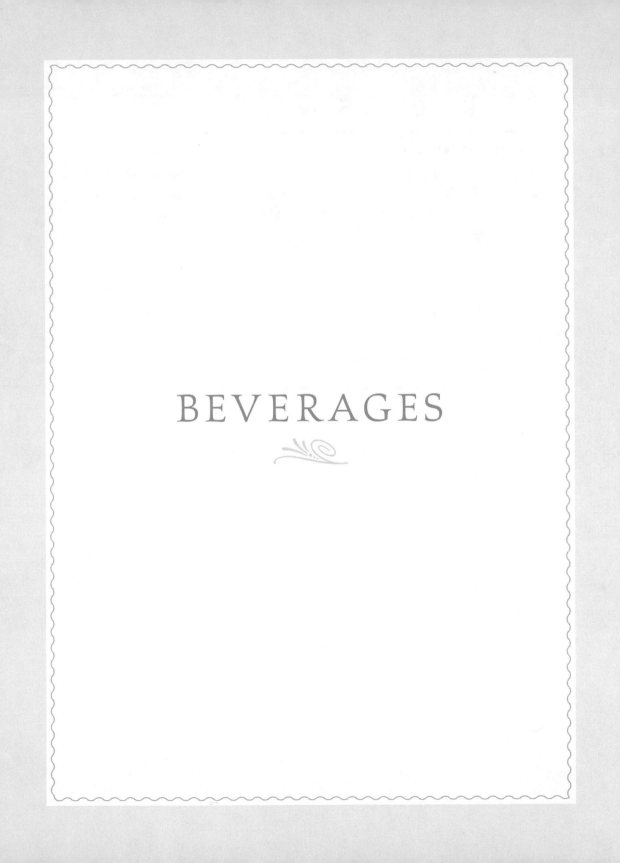

Berrylicious Tofu Smoothie

MAKES 2 SERVINGS

Tofu forms the base of this nutritious smoothie, giving it a creamy texture as well as a boost of protein to jump-start your day. Banana adds natural sweetness so no additional sugar is needed. This smoothie is rich in protein, fiber, calcium, and folate. It also has a full day's supply of Vitamin C!

1 package (10 ounces) frozen mixed berries
6 ounces (¾ cup) silken tofu
½ banana, frozen
¾ cup calcium-fortified orange juice

Blend all ingredients together in a blender on high speed until smooth.

NUTRITIONAL INFORMATION
One serving: Calories 195; Fat 3g (Sat 0.5g); Protein 7.5g; Carb 38g; Fiber 6.3g; Calcium 282mg; Iron 1.1mg; Sodium 15mg; Folate 60µg

Note: If using fresh berries or a room temperature banana instead of frozen, add a few ice cubes to the blender.

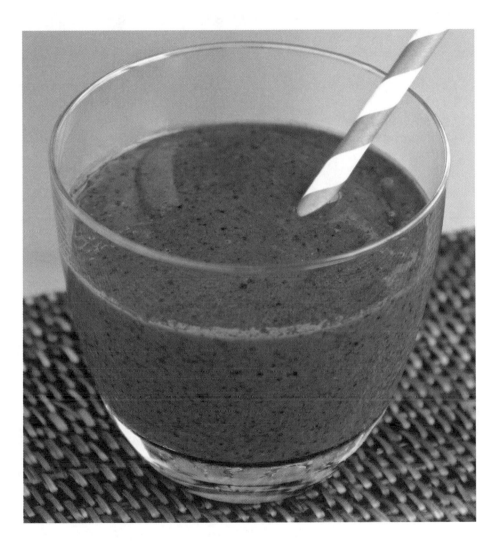

Nutty for Chocolate Banana Smoothie

MAKES 2 SERVINGS

This tasty smoothie will satisfy even the most serious chocolate cravings while also providing a variety of healthful nutrients! Wheat germ is an easy way to add a boost of protein, fiber, zinc, iron, and folate. This dish also provides plenty of calcium and Vitamin D.

1½ cups skim or low-fat milk
1 banana
2 tablespoons creamy peanut butter
1 tablespoon wheat germ or ground flaxseed

1½ tablespoons Nesquik® chocolate syrup or 3 tablespoons low sugar chocolate powder
¾ cup ice

Blend all ingredients together in a blender until smooth. Serve immediately.

NUTRITIONAL INFORMATION
One serving: Calories 292; Fat 8.5g (Sat 1.9g); Protein 13.9g; Carb 43.5g; Fiber 2.9g; Calcium 308mg; Iron 3.1mg; Sodium 200mg; Folate 119µg

Note: Nesquik® chocolate syrup does not use any high fructose corn syrup. The powder is fortified with several vitamins and minerals.

Mariya's Green Smoothie

MAKES 2 SERVINGS

This recipe was shared by my good friend Mariya, whom I first met in culinary school. When Mariya was pregnant, she developed an aversion to the leafy green veggies she used to enjoy. As a result, her husband (also a chef), started incorporating them into smoothies like this one. By combining spinach and kale with mango, strawberries, and watermelon, she was able to get her needed greens while enjoying a delicious and refreshing treat. This smoothie is chock full of nutrients, including folate and calcium. It also provides a good amount of protein and fiber for long-lasting energy.

1 cup spinach, packed
1 cup kale, packed
1 medium mango, peeled
1½ cups cubed watermelon, seeded
Juice of ½ lime

½ cup halved strawberries
¼ cup plain, reduced-fat Greek
   yogurt
¼ cup cold water

Steam the spinach and kale for 2 minutes. Drain, squeezing out any excess water. Place the greens in a blender along with all of the remaining ingredients. Blend on high speed until smooth. Serve.

NUTRITIONAL INFORMATION
One serving: Calories 188; Fat 1.5g (Sat 0.7g); Protein 6.8g; Carb 42.2g; Fiber 4.9g; Calcium 148mg; Iron 1.7mg; Sodium 37mg; Folate 126µg

Banana Nut Health Shake

MAKES 2 SERVINGS

Go nuts with this filling breakfast shake that features a double dose of almonds. It's packed with protein, fiber, omega-3 fatty acids, and whole grains that will give you long-lasting energy to kick-start your day. It also provides more than half of your daily calcium needs!

1 medium banana
2 cups fortified unsweetened vanilla
   almond milk
¾ cup old-fashioned oats
1½ tablespoons almond butter
1 tablespoon ground flaxseed or

flaxseed oil
¼ teaspoon vanilla extract
⅛ teaspoon cinnamon plus extra for
   garnish
2 tablespoons maple syrup
½ cup ice

Place all ingredients in a blender and blend until smooth. Garnish with cinnamon.

NUTRITIONAL INFORMATION
One serving: Calories 339; Fat 11.7g (Sat 1g); Protein 8.9g; Carb 50.8g; Fiber 6.6g; Calcium 538mg; Iron 2.6mg; Sodium 164mg; Folate 30µg

Mango Peach Blast

MAKES 2 SERVINGS

The vibrant yellow color and bright flavors in this smoothie will make you feel like you're vacationing on a tropical island. Greek yogurt adds a boost of protein and flaxseed provides plenty of omega-3s. This drink also provides a good amount of fiber, calcium, and folate, and more than half your daily supply of Vitamin C.

1 cup frozen diced mango
1 cup frozen sliced peaches
½ cup orange juice, plus additional as desired
½ cup low-fat or nonfat plain Greek yogurt

2 teaspoons honey or other sweetener
1 tablespoon ground flaxseed or flaxseed oil

Place all of the ingredients together in a blender and blend until smooth. Add additional orange juice or water as needed to thin out the smoothie. Pour into two glasses and serve.

NUTRITIONAL INFORMATION
One serving: Calories 191; Fat 3g (Sat 1.1g); Protein 8.2g; Carb 35.9g; Fiber 3.6g; Calcium 147mg; Iron 0.6mg; Sodium 21mg; Folate 52µg

Note: If using fresh fruit, add a few ice cubes to the blender.

Hydrating Honeydew Lemonade

MAKES 6 SERVINGS

Hydration is key in pregnancy but that doesn't mean that you have to limit yourself to plain water. This refreshing beverage combines freshly squeezed lemon juice with sweet honeydew to provide plenty of water and about half of your daily Vitamin C needs.

2 pounds honeydew melon (about
   ½ medium melon)
½ cup freshly squeezed lemon juice
2½ cups water
3 tablespoons honey or sweetener
   of your choice

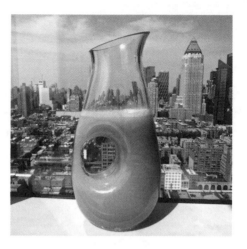

Peel and cube the honeydew and puree it in a blender. You should have about 2 cups of puree. Pour it into a pitcher along with the lemon juice, water, and sweetener. Stir to combine well. Taste and adjust sweetness to taste. Serve over ice.

NUTRITIONAL INFORMATION

One serving: Calories 90; Fat 0.2g (Sat 0.1g); Protein 0.9g; Carb 23.8g; Fiber 1.3g; Calcium 13mg; Iron 0.3mg; Sodium 31mg; Folate 32µg

---

Watermelon Agua Fresca

MAKES 6 SERVINGS

Living up to its name, watermelon is comprised of about 92 percent water. It's also full of important antioxidants, vitamins and electrolytes. Agua fresca, which means "fresh water," is a popular cold beverage in Mexico, Central America, and the Caribbean. It's made with a mixture of water and fruit and is the perfect rejuvenating drink, especially during hot summer months.

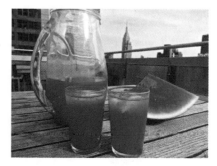

4 cups cubed watermelon

4 cups water, divided

2 tablespoons honey or other sweetener of your choice

2 tablespoons lime juice

Place the watermelon in a blender with 1 cup water, honey, and lime juice. Puree until smooth. Pour the mixture into a pitcher and add the remaining 3 cups water. Stir to combine. Refrigerate until cold. Serve over ice.

NUTRITIONAL INFORMATION

One serving: Calories 52; Fat 0.1g (Sat 0g); Protein 0.7g; Carb 13.8g; Fiber 0.4g; Calcium 12mg; Iron 0.3mg; Sodium 7mg; Folate 3µg

Baby Bellini

MAKES 4 SERVINGS

Created at a bar in Venice, Italy, the bellini is a classic cocktail made with peach puree and Prosecco, a sparkling wine. This virgin version uses sparkling apple cider, which provides plenty of Vitamin C. It's perfect to serve at parties, brunches, or even a baby shower. Take advantage of fresh peaches when in season, otherwise use frozen peaches or bottled peach nectar.

½ cup peach puree*

2 cups chilled sparkling cider

8 raspberries

Pour 2 tablespoons peach puree into four champagne flutes. Slowly pour ½ cup sparkling cider into each. Drop 2 raspberries into each glass and serve.

NUTRITIONAL INFORMATION

One serving: Calories 79; Fat 0.1g (Sat 0g); Protein 0.7g; Carb 20g; Fiber 0.5g; Calcium 1mg; Iron 0.1mg; Sodium 0mg; Folate 1µg

*To make peach puree, blend frozen peaches in a high-speed blender. If peaches are in season, use ripe, peeled peaches.

Pineapple Ginger Spritzer

MAKES 4 SERVINGS

Homemade fruit spritzers were my drink of choice during pregnancy. Simply pour your favorite fruit juice or puree over ice and top it off with some sparkling water for a fun and fizzy thirst-quencher. This easy drink provides plenty of water and Vitamin C and the ginger may help alleviate nausea.

2 cups pineapple juice
1-inch piece fresh ginger peeled and sliced
   (can substitute 1 tablespoon chopped crystallized ginger)
1 cup sparkling water or club soda

Place the pineapple juice and ginger in a saucepan and bring to a simmer. Remove from heat and transfer to a bowl. Cover and refrigerate overnight (or at least 8 hours).

Strain the juice and discard the ginger. Pour it into four glasses filled with ice. Top the glasses off with the sparkling water. Stir and serve.

NUTRITIONAL INFORMATION
One serving: Calories 67; Fat 0.1g (Sat 0g); Protein 0.5g; Carb 16.4g; Fiber 0.3g; Calcium 24mg; Iron 0.4mg; Sodium 3mg; Folate 22μg

Cucumber Faux-jito

MAKES 4 SERVINGS

Don't feel left out at parties—enjoy fun mocktails like this virgin mojito. It has all the flavors of a classic mojito like fresh mint and lime but substitutes cucumber juice for the rum. This tasty and incredibly refreshing drink will keep you hydrated and provide plenty of Vitamin C, Vitamin K, and potassium.

2 cups peeled, seeded and diced
  cucumber
20 mint leaves
1 lime, cut into wedges
4 teaspoons honey or other
  sweetener of choice

3 cups sparkling water or club soda
Cucumber slices for garnish

Place the cucumber in a blender and puree until smooth. You should have about one cup of puree.

Place 5-6 mint leaves and 1 lime wedge in the bottom of each of four glasses. Crush them with a muddler or the handle of a wooden spoon to release the flavors and juice. Add ¼ cup cucumber puree and 1 teaspoon honey to each glass and stir to combine. Fill the glasses with ice and add ¾ cup sparkling water or club soda to each glass. Add a few cucumber slices and serve.

NUTRITIONAL INFORMATION
One serving: Calories 34; Fat 0g (Sat 0g); Protein 0.6g; Carb 9.1g; Fiber 1g; Calcium 41mg; Iron 0.4mg; Sodium 3mg; Folate 11µg

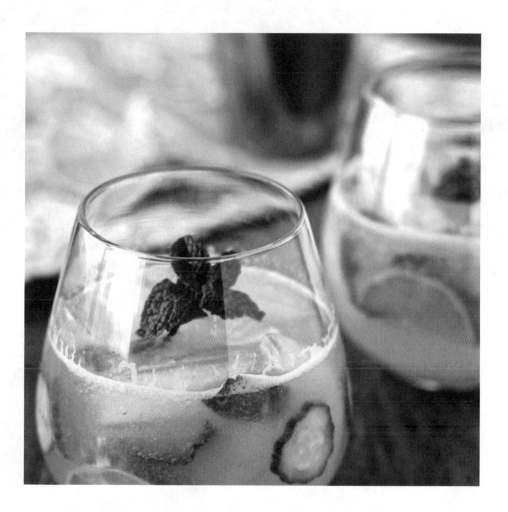

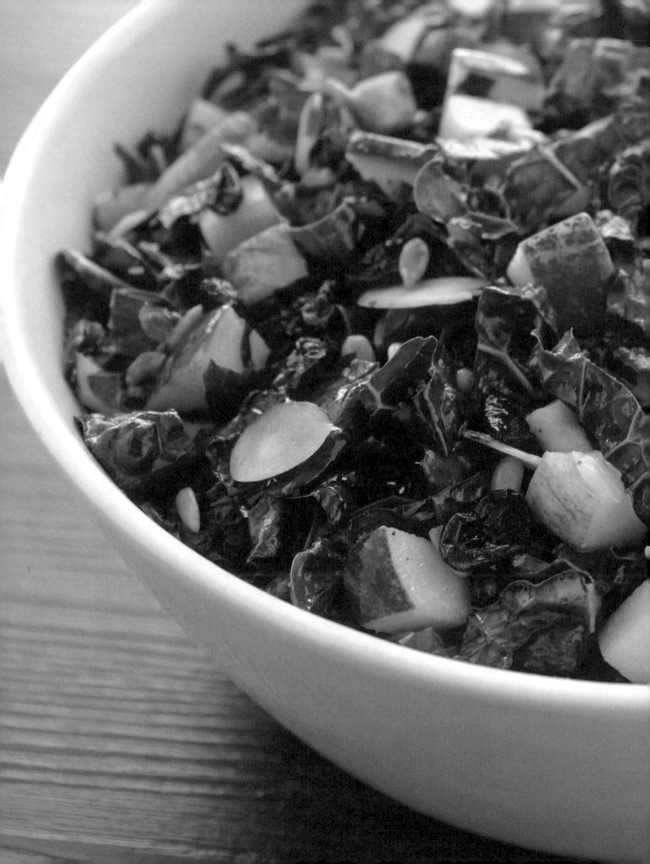

SOUPS, SALADS, AND DRESSINGS

Classic Chicken Noodle Soup

MAKES 4 SERVINGS

Recent studies show what mothers have known for generations—chicken soup may actually help you fight off a cold. Whether you're feeling a little under the weather or just want a comforting bowl of soup to warm you up, you can't beat this dish. It's packed with antioxidants, protein, fiber, iron, and folate. Homemade stock makes all the difference in a simple soup like this so try the recipe for Homemade Chicken Stock (page 147). If you're pressed for time, go for a high-quality packaged stock, preferably organic.

4 teaspoons olive oil
1 medium onion, chopped
3 garlic cloves, minced
2 medium carrots, peeled and cut into ½-inch-thick slices
2 celery ribs, cut into ½-inch-thick slices
2 fresh thyme sprigs
1 bay leaf
2 quarts Homemade Chicken Stock (see page 147) or packaged low-sodium chicken stock

5 ounces wide egg noodles (about 2½ cups)
8 ounces shredded cooked chicken (about 2 cups)
1 tablespoon fresh lemon juice
Kosher salt and freshly ground black pepper, to taste
¼ cup parsley, chopped

Place a large heavy-bottomed pot over medium heat and add the oil. Add the onion, garlic, carrots, celery, thyme and bay leaf. Cook until vegetables are softened, about 7 to 8 minutes. Pour in the chicken stock and bring the liquid to a boil. Lower to a simmer and cook for 5 minutes until vegetables are tender. Add the noodles and simmer another 6 to 7 minutes until cooked. Stir in the chicken and lemon juice and simmer another couple of minutes until heated through. Season the soup with salt and pepper to taste. Stir in the parsley. Serve hot.

NUTRITIONAL INFORMATION
One serving: Calories 376; Fat 10.8g (Sat 2.8g); Protein 31.1g; Carb 38.8g; Fiber 3.2g; Calcium 77mg; Iron 3.8mg; Sodium 231mg; Folate 159µg

Homemade Chicken Stock

MAKES 2 QUARTS

You can use this recipe as a base for many delicious soups and sauces, including Classic Chicken Noodle Soup (page 146). I usually double the recipe and store extra stock in the freezer.

- 1 whole (3–3½ pounds) chicken, preferably organic
- 1 medium onion, quartered
- 2 carrots, cut into large pieces
- 2 celery stalks, cut into large pieces
- 1 head garlic, unpeeled and cut in half crosswise

- 4 sprigs fresh thyme
- 10 sprigs parsley with stems
- 2 bay leaves
- 1 teaspoon kosher salt
- 1 teaspoon black peppercorns

Add all of the ingredients to a large heavy-bottomed pot or stockpot. Pour in enough cold water to just cover the chicken. Bring the liquid to a boil then reduce to a simmer. Simmer gently for 1 to 1½ hours, partially covered, until the chicken is cooked. As it simmers, skim off any impurities that rise to the surface.

Carefully remove the chicken with tongs and place it on a cutting board. Discard the skin and bones. Shred the meat and store it in the refrigerator in an airtight container.

Strain the stock through a fine sieve into another bowl. Cover and refrigerate. The next day, remove the surface fat. Store the stock in the refrigerator for up to 1 week or in the freezer for 3 months.

NUTRITIONAL INFORMATION
One cup: Calories 38; Fat 1g (Sat 0g); Protein 5g; Carb 3g; Fiber 0g; Calcium 9.6mg; Iron 0.5mg; Sodium 72mg; Folate 0µg

Comfort in a Bowl Carrot Ginger Soup

MAKES 4 SERVINGS

Is there anything more comforting than a warm bowl of soup? This creamy soup is packed with flavor and nutrients, thanks to carrots. Their rich orange color means they're packed with beta-carotene, which gets converted to Vitamin A in the body and is essential for vision, immune health, growth, and reproduction. This hearty soup also provides a good amount of fiber, calcium, folate, and Vitamin C. Ginger may help alleviate morning sickness.

1½ tablespoons olive oil
1 medium yellow onion, chopped
1 tablespoon minced ginger
2 cloves garlic, minced
1½ teaspoons ground coriander
1½ pounds carrots, peeled and
    chopped

4 cups vegetable (or chicken) stock
¼ cup freshly squeezed orange juice
¼ cup reduced-fat or nonfat plain
    Greek yogurt
Salt and pepper, to taste
Cilantro leaves for garnish (optional)

Heat the oil in a large Dutch oven or other soup pot over medium heat. Add the onion and cook until just softened, about 5 to 6 minutes. Stir in the ginger, garlic, and coriander and cook for another minute until fragrant. Add the carrots and vegetable stock. Bring to a boil then reduce heat to a simmer and cover the pot. Cook until carrots are tender, about 20 minutes. Stir in the orange juice.

Using an immersion blender, carefully puree the soup until smooth. Alternatively, you can puree the soup in a blender, working in batches if necessary. Season the soup with salt and pepper to taste. To serve, ladle the soup into four bowls and top each with a dollop of yogurt. Garnish with cilantro, if desired.

NUTRITIONAL INFORMATION
One serving: Calories 161; Fat 5.7g (Sat 1g); Protein 3.3g; Carb 26.1g; Fiber 5.6g; Calcium 108mg; Iron 0.8mg; Sodium 204mg; Folate 43µg

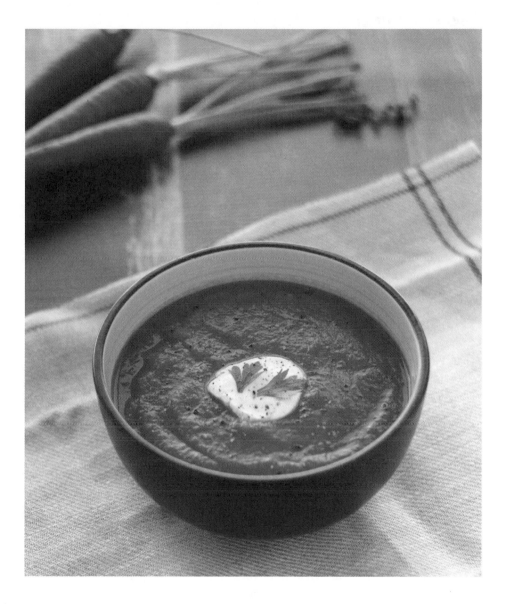

Italian Lentil Soup

MAKES 6 SERVINGS

This recipe was shared by my wonderful mother-in-law who stopped eating meat when she was pregnant with my husband. At the time, she thought it was just a temporary aversion but to this day, she's remained a vegetarian. This is the kind of soup you'll want to curl up with on a cold winter's day. Lentils are an excellent vegetarian source of protein and fiber, which will keep you feeling full and satisfied. This dish is also rich in iron and folate.

1 tablespoon olive oil plus extra for drizzling
1 medium onion, chopped
1 medium carrot, peeled and chopped
2 stalks celery, chopped
2 cloves garlic, minced
1 can (6 ounces) tomato paste
1½ cups brown lentils, rinsed and drained

8 cups water
1 teaspoon dried basil
2 teaspoons kosher salt
6 ounces (about 1½ cups) ditalini pasta
Optional: grated Parmigiano-Reggiano cheese for serving

Heat 1 tablespoon olive oil over medium heat in a large Dutch oven or other heavy-bottomed pot. Add the onion, carrot, and celery and cook until onion is transparent, about 6 to 8 minutes. Add the garlic and sauté for an additional 1 to 2 minutes. Add the tomato paste, lentils, water, basil, and salt. Bring all ingredients to a boil, reduce heat to simmer, cover and cook until lentils are tender, about 30 minutes.

Add the pasta and cook until al dente, about 10 minutes. Test the lentils and pasta to make sure they are done. Taste and adjust seasoning as desired. Serve with a drizzle of olive oil and grated cheese.

NUTRITIONAL INFORMATION
One serving: Calories 245; Fat 4.8g (Sat 0.7g); Protein 13.2g; Carb 47.3g; Fiber 11.7g; Calcium 41mg; Iron 2.1mg; Sodium 839mg; Folate 121µg

White Gazpacho

MAKES 4 SERVINGS

Soup isn't just for cold weather. A refreshing bowl of cold soup can be the perfect thirst-quencher on a hot summer day. White gazpacho originates from Spain and is made by pureeing heart-healthy olive oil and almonds with water-dense cucumbers and grapes. This rejuvenating soup will keep you hydrated and provide protein, folate, and several other vitamins and minerals.

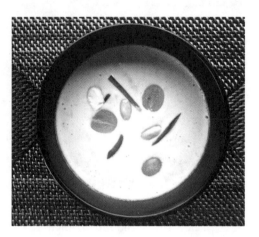

2.5 ounces cubed white bread (about 2 cups) from a baguette, Italian loaf or sliced bread (crust cut off)

1½ cups cold water, divided

⅓ cup whole, blanched almonds

1 clove garlic

2 tablespoons chopped shallot

2 cups diced, peeled English cucumber (about 1 large cucumber)

¾ cup green grapes

2 tablespoons extra virgin olive oil

3½ teaspoons sherry vinegar

1 teaspoon kosher salt

Chives or scallions for garnish (optional)

Place the bread cubes in a bowl and pour ½ cup water on top to soften them. Place the almonds and garlic in a blender and puree until finely ground. Add the shallot, cucumber, grapes, oil, vinegar, salt and softened bread to the blender, along with the remaining 1 cup water. Puree until smooth. Taste and adjust salt as needed.

Add more water to the soup as needed to achieve desired consistency. Serve at room temperature or chilled. Serve in bowls or glasses and garnish with sliced grapes, almonds and chives or scallions if desired.

NUTRITIONAL INFORMATION

One serving: Calories 210; Fat 13.1g (Sat 1.6g); Protein 4.7g; Carb 19g; Fiber 2.4g; Calcium 73mg; Iron 1.4mg; Sodium 679mg; Folate 47µg

---

Roasted Eggplant and Tomato Soup with Fresh Herbs

MAKES 2 SERVINGS

Pureed soups like this are a great way to get in a lot of healthful veggies, especially on days when you're not feeling up to eating much. This recipe was shared by my friend Ann over at Sumptuous Spoonfuls (www.sumptuousspoonfuls.com). Ann is an engineer as well as a fantastic cook and has a wonderful site with a collection of eclectic, healthy and delicious recipes. As she describes it, red tomatoes give this soup an enticing hue that pulls you into the bowl. Eggplant lends a delightful creaminess and buttery taste. This dish is packed with protein, fiber, calcium, iron, and folate.

½ medium eggplant (8 ounces), peeled and sliced into ½-inch slices

½ medium yellow onion, peeled and cut into large chunks

4 cloves garlic, peeled

1½ tablespoons olive oil, divided

4 medium ripe tomatoes (24 ounces), sliced in half

2 cups low-sodium chicken or vegetable broth

1 bay leaf

2 tablespoons fresh herbs (thyme, rosemary, oregano, basil, tarragon) plus extra for garnish

½ cup whole milk or half and half (optional)

2 tablespoons crumbled pasteurized goat cheese (or feta)

Salt and pepper, to taste

Preheat the oven to 400°F. Place the eggplant slices, onion, and garlic on a baking sheet and brush them with 1 tablespoon oil. Place the tomatoes on a second baking sheet and toss them with the remaining ½ tablespoon oil. Arrange the tomatoes in a single layer, cut side down.

Roast all of the vegetables in the oven for 15 to 20 minutes until tender and brown in spots. Roast the tomatoes for an additional 10 minutes. Carefully remove the tomato skins with tongs (they should pull off easily).

Place the roasted vegetables and tomatoes (with juices) in a large saucepan and add the broth, bay leaf, and herbs. Bring to a boil then reduce heat to a simmer. Simmer until vegetables are tender and broth is partially reduced, about 20 minutes.

Cool slightly. Remove the bay leaf. Transfer the soup to a blender and puree until smooth. Return to the soup to the saucepan and stir in the milk, if using. Season the soup with salt and pepper to taste.

Ladle the hot soup into bowls, sprinkle with some goat cheese, and garnish with fresh herbs. Serve with toasted bread to mop up every drop.

NUTRITIONAL INFORMATION
One serving: Calories 277; Fat 14.9g (Sat 4.1g); Protein 12.4g; Carb 28.3g; Fiber 9g; Calcium 102mg; Iron 2.7mg; Sodium 145mg; Folate 85µg

---

Power-Packed Pasta Fagioli

MAKES 8 SERVINGS

Pasta fagioli is a classic Italian soup with humble peasant origins. Made from inexpensive ingredients like pasta and beans, this dish is full of flavor, while also being satisfying and healthy. To boost the nutrition even more, I like to add some chopped kale, a super food. This dish is packed with protein, fiber, iron, calcium, and folate.

1 tablespoon olive oil
2 ounces pancetta, diced (optional)
1 medium yellow onion, diced
2 large carrots, peeled and diced
2 stalks celery, diced
3 cloves garlic, minced
¼ teaspoon red pepper flakes
1½ teaspoons chopped, fresh rosemary or ½ teaspoon dried
1 bay leaf
1 can (14.5 ounces) crushed tomatoes
2 quarts low-sodium chicken or vegetable broth

2 cans (15.5 ounces) cannellini (white kidney) beans, drained and rinsed
1½ cups small pasta like ditalini or elbows (preferably whole grain)
5 ounces (1 bunch) chopped kale leaves
2 tablespoons grated Parmigiano-Reggiano cheese (plus extra for garnish)
Salt and pepper, to taste

Heat the oil in a large Dutch oven or other heavy bottomed pot over medium heat. Add the pancetta (if using) and cook for a couple of minutes until it starts to brown. Add the onion, carrots, and celery and cook, stirring occasionally, until partially softened, about 5 to 6 minutes. Add the garlic, red pepper flakes, rosemary, and bay leaf and cook for another minute until fragrant. Add the tomatoes and chicken broth and raise the heat to bring to a simmer.

Place about a quarter cup of beans in a bowl and add a little bit of the cooking liquid. Mash them together to form a paste and add it to the pot, along with the rest of the whole beans. Simmer the soup uncovered for 15 minutes and then add the pasta. Simmer another 10 minutes until pasta is tender and then add the kale. Cook for 5 minutes until kale is wilted. Stir in the cheese. Season with salt and pepper

Ladle the soup into bowls and top with grated cheese, if desired. Soup will thicken as it stands.

NUTRITIONAL INFORMATION
One serving: Calories 277; Fat 4.7g (Sat 1.3g); Protein 17g; Carb 44.2g; Fiber 8.9g; Calcium 113mg; Iron 3.8mg; Sodium 490mg; Folate 120µg

---

Tuscan Kale and Apple Salad

MAKES 4 SERVINGS

Salads don't have to be boring! This lovely fall salad combines contrasting flavors and textures in a visually stunning dish that will make you want to dive right in. Kale is a nutritional superstar that can be eaten raw or cooked. I like to use Tuscan kale in this dish since the leaves are more tender and milder in flavor than curly kale. You'll pretty much get it all with this dish—healthy fats (including omega-3s), protein, fiber, antioxidants, and several important vitamins and minerals.

Salad
1 bunch (10 ounces) Tuscan (also called Lacinato) kale
1 medium apple like Fuji or Honeycrisp, diced
2 tablespoons reduced-sugar dried cranberries

4 teaspoons sunflower seeds
2 tablespoons sliced almonds
1 ounce firm cheese like Piave, Parmigiano-Reggiano or Manchego, shaved with a vegetable peeler

Dressing

1 tablespoon cider vinegar

1 teaspoon Dijon mustard

1 teaspoon honey

2 tablespoons extra virgin olive oil

Salt and pepper, to taste

To make the dressing, whisk the vinegar, mustard, honey, and oil together in a small bowl. Season with salt and pepper.

To make the salad, remove the kale leaves from the stems and discard the stems. Slice the leaves thinly (you should have about 5 cups). Place the kale in a salad bowl and add the dressing. Massage the dressing into the kale, coating all of the leaves well. This will help the kale absorb the dressing and also help tenderize the leaves. Add the apple, dried cranberries, sunflower seeds, and almonds and toss to combine. Sprinkle the cheese on top and serve.

NUTRITIONAL INFORMATION
One serving: Calories 206; Fat 11.8g (Sat 2.5g); Protein 6.5g; Carb 20.7g; Fiber 3.7g; Calcium 208mg; Iron 1.9mg; Sodium 181mg; Folate 33mg

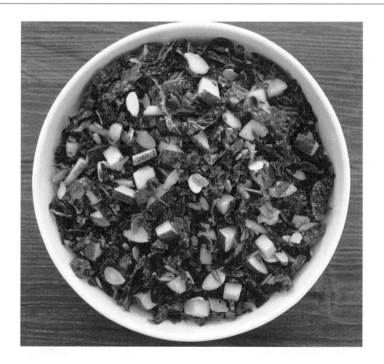

Butter Lettuce Salad with Buttermilk Herb Dressing

MAKES 4 SERVINGS

This vibrant salad screams summer. Delicate butter lettuce, luscious heirloom tomatoes, and grilled, sweet corn are drizzled with a homemade buttermilk ranch dressing. This salad provides antioxidants, fiber, and several vitamins and minerals including B vitamins, folate, and Vitamin C.

1 teaspoon olive oil
2 ears corn, shucked
Kosher salt
1 head butter lettuce, leaves separated
2 heirloom tomatoes, cut into wedges

Buttermilk Herb Dressing (see page 156)
Fresh herbs (parsley, dill, chives) for garnish

Heat a grill pan over medium high heat. Rub the olive oil on the corn and season with salt. Grill the corn, turning occasionally, until cooked, about 8 to 10 minutes. Let the corn cool and then cut the kernels from the cobs.

Arrange the lettuce on a serving platter. Top with the tomatoes and corn. Drizzle Buttermilk Herb Dressing on top. Garnish with fresh herbs.

NUTRITIONAL INFORMATION
One serving: Calories 69; Fat 1.9g (Sat 0.4g); Protein 2.8g; Carb 12.8g; Fiber 2.2g; Calcium 21mg; Iron 0.9mg; Sodium 12mg; Folate 59mg

Buttermilk Herb Dressing

MAKES ABOUT 2 CUPS DRESSING

Store-bought salad dressings often have a lot of added sugars, preservatives, and a surprising number of calories. This versatile homemade dressing is like a cross between ranch and green goddess dressings and can also double as a dip. A combination of reduced-fat buttermilk and Greek yogurt allows you to cut back on the amount of mayonnaise while also adding a boost of protein.

1 cup reduced-fat buttermilk	2 tablespoons chives
⅔ cup nonfat or reduced-fat Greek yogurt	1 tablespoon dill
	1½ tablespoons lemon juice
¼ cup reduced-fat mayonnaise	1 small clove garlic
1 teaspoon Dijon mustard	Salt and pepper, to taste
2 tablespoons parsley	

Blend all ingredients together in a blender until smooth. Season with salt and pepper to taste. Store in the refrigerator.

NUTRITIONAL INFORMATION
One serving (2 tablespoons): Calories 15; Fat 0.3g (Sat 0.1g); Protein 1.6g; Carb 1.5g; Fiber 0.1g; Calcium 25mg; Iron 0.1mg; Sodium 29mg; Folate 2mg

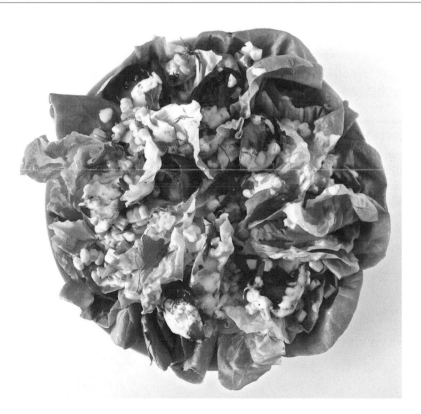

Chicken Salad with a Twist

MAKES 4 SERVINGS

I created this dish when I was looking for something to spice up my chicken salad recipe. I found a bottle of za'atar in my spice drawer and this recipe was born. Za'atar is a versatile Middle Eastern spice blend that can be used on meats, veggies, rice, and bread. This dish provides plenty of protein and iron. I like to serve it on toasted whole grain bread with some baby spinach for an extra boost of nutrition.

3 cups cooked, diced chicken breast (12 ounces)
½ cup sliced celery
½ cup red grapes, halved
3 tablespoons sliced almonds
¼ cup Homemade Vegan Mayonnaise (see page 123) or reduced-fat mayonnaise

2 tablespoons nonfat or reduced-fat Greek yogurt
¾ teaspoon za'atar (optional)
Salt and pepper, to taste

Place the chicken, celery, grapes, and almonds in a large bowl. Mix the mayonnaise and yogurt together and add it to the ingredients in the bowl. Add the za'atar and season with salt and pepper to taste. Stir to combine.

NUTRITIONAL INFORMATION
One serving: Calories 264; Fat 9.5g (Sat 1.7g); Protein 36.1g; Carb 5.9g; Fiber 1.3g; Calcium 72mg; Iron 2mg; Sodium 143mg; Folate 14mg

Za'atar is a Middle Eastern dried spice mix with sumac, sesame seeds, and other spices like oregano and thyme.

Quinoa Salad with Spinach, Strawberries, and Goat Cheese

MAKES 4 SERVINGS

Quinoa is a pregnancy super food! This whole grain is packed with protein, fiber, and several vitamins and minerals including iron, folate and manganese. This salad pairs red quinoa with fresh spinach (another super food), sweet strawberries, tangy goat cheese, and crunchy almonds, all tossed with a simple balsamic vinaigrette. As an added bonus, the Vitamin C in the strawberries will help your body absorb the iron in the quinoa.

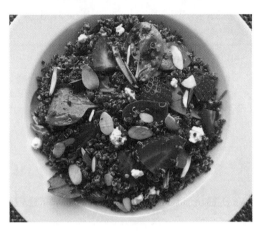

1 cup red quinoa (can substitute white)
2 cups baby spinach leaves
2 tablespoons fresh basil, cut into chiffonade (ribbons)
⅔ cup sliced strawberries

1 ounce pasteurized goat cheese, crumbled
1½ tablespoons sliced almonds, toasted
Kosher salt, to taste

Balsamic Dressing

2 tablespoons balsamic vinegar
1 teaspoon Dijon mustard
½ teaspoon honey

2 tablespoons extra virgin olive oil
Kosher salt and black pepper, to taste

Place the quinoa in a medium saucepan along with 2 cups water and ¼ teaspoon salt. Bring to a boil, and then cover with a lid and reduce to a simmer. Simmer the quinoa for about 15 minutes until cooked. Remove the lid and cook for another 2 to 3 minutes until all of the water has evaporated. Remove from the heat and fluff with a fork. Let the quinoa cool to room temperature.

Meanwhile, make the balsamic dressing. Whisk the vinegar, mustard, and honey together in a small bowl. Slowly pour in the olive oil while you continue to whisk. Season the dressing with salt and pepper.

Place the quinoa in a salad bowl along with the spinach, basil, strawberries, goat cheese, and almonds. Add the dressing and toss to combine all ingredients well. Serve the salad alone or, if desired, topped with slices of grilled chicken breast.

NUTRITIONAL INFORMATION
One serving: Calories 271; Fat 11.6g (Sat 2.4g); Protein 8.5g; Carb 32.6g; Fiber 4g; Calcium 58mg; Iron 2.8mg; Sodium 73mg; Folate 116mg

---

Roasted Butternut Squash Salad with Maple Dijon Vinaigrette

MAKES 4 SERVINGS

This delicious fall salad features butternut squash, which is rich in flavor and nutrients. Roasted cubes of squash are tossed with a mixture of greens, dried cranberries, and a homemade vinaigrette that's sweetened with maple syrup. Heart-healthy pecans add crunch and goat cheese (use pasteurized) adds a salty bite. This salad is rich in protein, fiber, calcium, iron, and folate.

½ medium butternut squash, peeled and cut into ¾-inch cubes (about 2½ cups)

1 teaspoon fresh thyme leaves, chopped (or ¼ teaspoon dried thyme)

2 tablespoons (6 teaspoons) extra virgin olive oil, divided use

¼ cup chopped pecans

1 tablespoon cider vinegar

1 tablespoon maple syrup

½ teaspoon Dijon mustard

2½ ounces (½ bag) baby arugula

2½ ounces (½ bag) baby spinach

¼ cup dried cranberries

2 ounces pasteurized goat cheese, crumbled

Kosher salt and black pepper, to taste

Preheat oven to 425°F. Toss the butternut squash with the thyme and 1 teaspoon olive oil on a baking sheet. Season the squash with salt and pepper and spread it out in a single layer. Roast in the oven for 20 minutes, then flip the squash over and cook another 10 minutes until fork tender. Turn the oven down to 350°F. Spread the pecans on a baking sheet and toast in the oven until fragrant, about 6 to 8 minutes. Remove from oven.

While the squash and pecans are cooking, whisk the vinegar, maple syrup, mustard, and remaining 5 teaspoons olive oil together in a small bowl. Season the vinaigrette with salt and pepper. Place the arugula and spinach in a salad bowl and toss with the dressing. Arrange the roasted squash, pecans, cranberries, and goat cheese on top.

NUTRITIONAL INFORMATION
One serving: Calories 230; Fat 14.4g (Sat 3.5g); Protein 5.1g; Carb 22.3g; Fiber 3.5g; Calcium 119mg; Iron 1.9mg; Sodium 90mg; Folate 77mg

Couscous Lentil Salad

MAKES 12 SERVINGS

This recipe was shared by my friend Christie, the inspirational woman behind Food Done Light (www.fooddonelight.com). Christie is an avid cook and self-proclaimed "food geek" and she shares her delicious and healthy recipes on her popular blog. This salad is packed with colorful grilled vegetables, fluffy couscous, and hearty lentils, which are an excellent source of complex carbohydrates, protein, fiber, and iron. This dish, which is satisfying enough to serve as a vegetarian entrée, also provides plenty of Vitamin C and folate.

¾ cup couscous, preferably whole wheat
8 mini red peppers or 1 large red pepper
1½ zucchini, sliced into planks
1 onion, cut into thick slices

1 teaspoon olive oil
½ teaspoon kosher salt
1 cup brown lentils, cooked
1 cup chopped cucumber
¼ cup chopped green onion
¼ cup chopped cilantro

Dressing
2 cloves garlic, chopped
2 tablespoons tahini paste
6 tablespoons lemon juice

¼ teaspoon kosher salt
½ cup buttermilk

Boil ¾ cup water and pour over couscous. Cover with plastic wrap and let sit for 5 minutes. Fluff couscous with a fork.

In a large bowl, toss red peppers, zucchini, and onion with the olive oil and salt. Heat a grill or grill pan to high heat and grill the vegetables for a minute or two on each side. Transfer to a cutting board and chop.

In a small food processor, puree all the ingredients for the dressing. Add the cooked lentils and grilled vegetables to the cooked couscous. Stir in the cucumber, green onion, and cilantro. Pour the dressing over the salad and toss well to combine.

NUTRITIONAL INFORMATION
One serving: Calories 150; Fat 2.2g (Sat 0.5g); Protein 8.4g; Carb 24.7g; Fiber 6.3g; Calcium 85mg; Iron 1.7mg; Sodium 177mg; Folate 99mg

Tropical Shrimp Salad

MAKES 6 SERVINGS

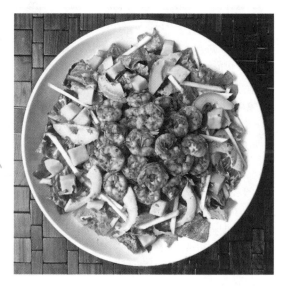

This light and refreshing salad has a tasty combination of sweet and spicy flavors. Fiery grilled shrimp are served on a bed of lettuce and tropical ingredients like mango, avocado, and jicama, which provide several important nutrients. Jicama is a crispy root vegetable native to Mexico that can be eaten raw or cooked. If you can't find it, you can substitute a firm pear or apple. This dish is packed with protein, fiber, Vitamin C, calcium, iron, and folate. Shrimp also add healthy omega-3 fatty acids.

Marinade

1 tablespoon olive oil
½ teaspoon ground cumin
1–2 teaspoons minced chipotles in adobo (depending on how spicy you like it)

2 teaspoons lime juice
2 cloves garlic, minced
1 pound large shrimp, peeled and deveined
Salt and pepper, to taste

Dressing

2 teaspoons Dijon mustard
1 teaspoon adobo sauce from the chipotle can
1 tablespoon honey

4 teaspoons lime juice
3 tablespoons olive oil
1 tablespoon chopped cilantro
Salt and pepper, to taste

Salad

1 head Romaine lettuce, chopped
1 mango, peeled and diced into cubes
1 medium jicama, peeled and julienned (cut into matchsticks)

1 avocado, peeled and sliced
2 tablespoons chopped cilantro

To make the marinade, pour the oil, cumin, chipotles, lime juice, and garlic into a large resealable plastic storage bag. Add the shrimp, seal the bag, and mix all of the ingredients together to coat the shrimp with the marinade. Let the shrimp marinate while you prepare the rest of the salad ingredients.

To make the dressing, whisk the mustard, adobo sauce, honey, lime juice, olive oil, and cilantro together in a bowl. Season the dressing with salt and pepper.

Heat a grill pan over medium high heat and spray with nonstick cooking spray. Season the shrimp with salt and pepper and add them to the grill. Cook for 2 to 3 minutes on each side until opaque.

To plate the salad, toss the lettuce, mango, and jicama with enough dressing to just coat all of the greens. Top the salad with the shrimp and arrange the avocado slices around them. Drizzle any remaining dressing on top and garnish with cilantro.

NUTRITIONAL INFORMATION
One serving: Calories 300, Fat 14.3g (Sat 2.2g); Protein 13.8g; Carb 29.3g; Fiber 11.1g; Calcium 102mg; Iron 2.3mg; Sodium 525mg; Folate 221mg

Lemon-Basil Three Bean Salad

MAKES 4 CUPS OR 8 SERVINGS

This satisfying vegetarian salad was shared by my friend Carrie at Carrie's Experimental Kitchen (www.carriesexperimentalkitchen.com). Looking to incorporate more beans into her diet, she developed this dish, which uses three different varieties of beans. Beans and other legumes are a fantastic vegetarian source of protein and are also packed with plenty of fiber, which is important for your digestive health. This dish is also rich in iron and folate.

1 can (15 ounces) black beans, rinsed
1 can (15 ounces) kidney beans, rinsed
1 can (15 ounces) chickpeas, rinsed
¼ cup red onion, chopped

¼ cup fresh basil, chopped
1 lemon, zest and juice
¼ cup white balsamic vinegar
¼ cup extra virgin olive oil
Kosher salt and black pepper, to taste

Combine all ingredients in a bowl and mix well. Season with salt and pepper to taste. Refrigerate until ready to serve.

NUTRITIONAL INFORMATION
One serving: Calories 212; Fat 7.6g (Sat 1g); Protein 8.8g; Carb 27.4g; Fiber 8.9g; Calcium 58mg; Iron 2.5mg; Sodium 315mg; Folate 89mg

Farro Salad with Corn, Tomatoes, and Edamame

MAKES 6 SERVINGS

This whole grain salad features farro, an ancient Italian grain with a nutty earthiness and satisfying chew. Farro is packed with important pregnancy nutrients like fiber, protein, B vitamins, folate, iron, and zinc. Use it in soups, casseroles, or hearty salads like this one. To maximize flavor, toss the dressing with the farro while it's still warm so that it fully absorbs it.

1 cup farro
4 cups water
1 clove garlic, smashed
1½ cups cooked corn
8 ounces grape tomatoes, halved
  (about 1½ cups)

1½ cups edamame, cooked
⅓ cup chopped parsley
1 ounce pasteurized feta cheese,
  crumbled
Salt, to taste

Sherry Vinaigrette
2 tablespoons sherry vinegar
2 tablespoons extra virgin olive oil
½ teaspoon Dijon mustard

¼ teaspoon kosher salt
⅛ teaspoon black pepper

Place the farro, water, and garlic in a medium saucepan. Season the water with salt and bring to a boil. Reduce heat to a simmer, cover, and cook until farro is done, about 25 to 30 minutes. Drain.

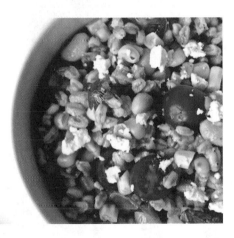

Meanwhile, make the sherry vinaigrette. Place the vinegar, oil, mustard, salt, and pepper together in a small jar or other container with a lid. Cover and shake until combined. Alternatively, you can whisk the ingredients together in a bowl.

Stir the warm farro together with the vinaigrette, corn, tomatoes, edamame, and parsley in a large bowl. Adjust seasoning to taste. Sprinkle cheese on top. Serve salad warm or chilled.

NUTRITIONAL INFORMATION
One serving: Calories 378; Fat 9g (Sat 1.9g); Protein 12.6g; Carb 62.7g; Fiber 10.8g; Calcium 74mg; Iron 3.2mg; Sodium 189mg; Folate 148mg

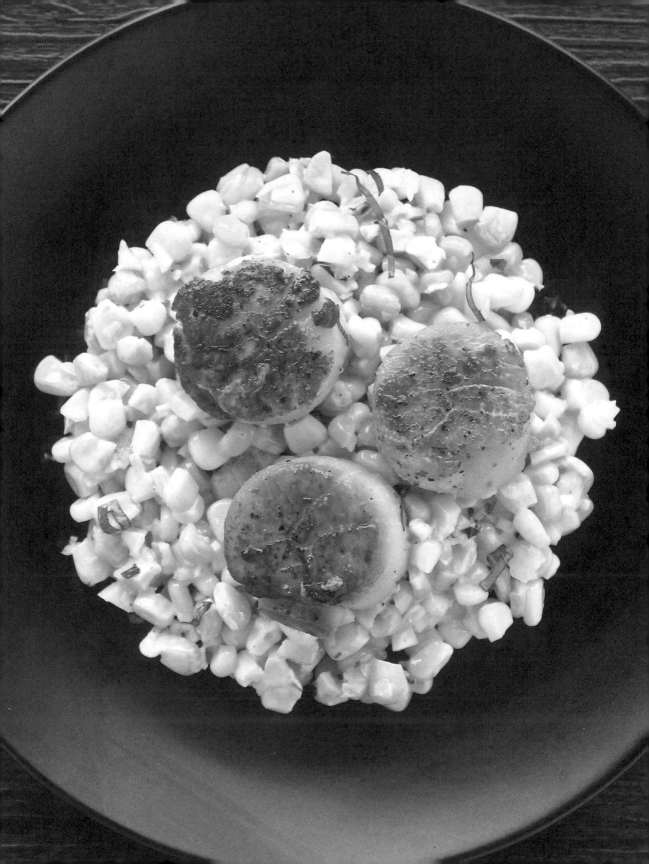

ENTRÉES

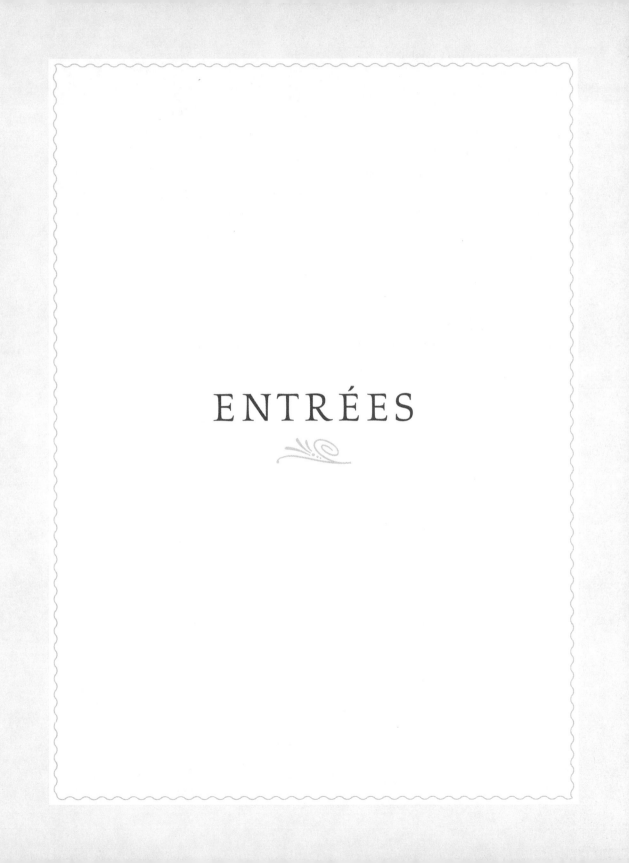

Quick and Easy Miso-Glazed Salmon

MAKES 4 SERVINGS

This is a quick and easy version of the classic miso glazed black cod made famous by Chef Nobu Matsuhisa at his NY restaurant Nobu. While the original dish requires three days of marinating, this version takes only 15 minutes from start to finish! Miso is a fermented soybean paste that forms a deliciously sticky-sweet glaze, coating the fish as it cooks. I like to use salmon as it's one of the most concentrated food sources of omega-3 fatty acids, but you can use any type of fish. This dish is also rich in protein, B vitamins, and several minerals.

4 (5-ounce) wild salmon fillets

2 tablespoons white (shiro) miso paste

1 tablespoon light soy sauce

4 teaspoons honey

Preheat the broiler. Place the salmon fillets in a shallow baking dish coated with cooking spray. Mix the miso paste, soy sauce, and honey together in a small bowl. Spoon the glaze evenly over the fillets.

Broil the salmon in the oven until cooked through, about 10 minutes. Baste the fish with the glaze halfway through. Serve immediately.

NUTRITIONAL INFORMATION

One serving: Calories 241; Fat 8.5g (Sat 1.5g); Protein 29.4g; Carb 8.4g; Fiber 0.5g; Calcium 22mg; Iron 1.5mg; Sodium 516mg; Folate 37µg

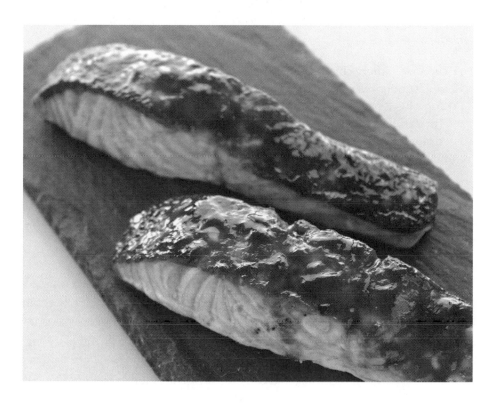

Tilapia Piccata

MAKES 4 SERVINGS

This simple yet elegant dish, which only takes about 20 minutes from start to finish, is a staple in my house. Classically made with chicken, this version uses tilapia and is a great way to incorporate seafood into your diet. To cut down on the amount of butter in the lemon butter sauce, I use flour, which thickens the sauce nicely. This dish will provide you with plenty of protein; B vitamins; and several minerals, like selenium, phosphorus, and potassium.

1 cup low-sodium chicken stock
1 tablespoon fresh lemon juice
¼ cup plus 2 teaspoons flour (preferably white whole wheat), divided use
4 tilapia fillets (about 5 ounces each)
1½ tablespoons olive oil

1 clove garlic, minced
2 tablespoons capers, drained
2 teaspoons unsalted butter
¼ cup parsley, chopped plus extra for garnish
Kosher salt and black pepper, to taste

Whisk the chicken stock, lemon juice and 2 teaspoons flour together in a measuring cup. Set aside.

Season the tilapia with salt and pepper. Place the remaining ¼ cup flour on a plate and lightly dredge the fillets in the flour on both sides, dusting off any excess. Discard the extra flour. Heat the oil in a large skillet over medium high heat and add the fish. Cook until golden, about 3 minutes, then carefully flip the filets over and cook another 3 minutes on the second side. Remove the fish and place on a plate.

Add the garlic to the skillet and cook for 30 seconds until fragrant. Pour the chicken stock mixture and capers into the skillet and cook until the sauce thickens, about 2 to 3 minutes. Lower the heat and stir in the butter and parsley. Return the tilapia fillets back to the pan and spoon the sauce over them. Cook another minute until warmed through. Garnish with extra parsley before serving.

NUTRITIONAL INFORMATION
One serving: Calories 229; Fat 9.2g (Sat 2.9g); Protein 30.5g; Carb 5.7g; Fiber 0.4g; Calcium 25mg; Iron 1.5mg; Sodium 221mg; Folate 56µg

Shrimp and Sausage Jambalaya

MAKES 4 SERVINGS

This classic New Orleans dish is chock full of flavor and nutrients! Shrimp add plenty of protein as well as brain-boosting omega-3s. Smoked turkey sausage is a lighter alternative to the classically used Andouille sausage. Brown rice is not traditional but using this whole grain adds B vitamins, fiber, and iron. Your whole family will love this delicious one-pot meal. Grab a fork and dig in!

1 tablespoon olive oil
8 ounces smoked turkey sausage (cooked), sliced into ¼-inch rounds
1 medium yellow onion, chopped
1 red or orange bell pepper, chopped
3 stalks celery, chopped
3 garlic cloves, chopped
1 tablespoon tomato paste
1 bay leaf
2 teaspoons chopped, fresh thyme or ¾ tsp dried thyme

½ teaspoon dried oregano
¼ teaspoon cayenne pepper
1 can (14.5 ounces) diced fire-roasted tomatoes
1¼ cups brown rice
3 cups low-sodium chicken broth or water
¾ pound large shrimp, peeled and deveined
1 tablespoon lemon juice
4 scallions, sliced
Hot sauce for serving (optional)
Salt and pepper, to taste

Heat the oil in a large Dutch oven or heavy-based pot. Add the sausage and brown on both sides, about 3 to 4 minutes. Add the onion, peppers, and celery and season them with salt and pepper. Cook for 5 to 6 minutes until they start to soften and then stir in the garlic and tomato paste. Cook another 2 minutes, and then add the bay leaf, thyme, oregano, and cayenne. Stir in the tomatoes, rice, and chicken broth.

Taste the liquid and season it with salt and pepper to taste. Bring the liquid to a boil, and then lower to a simmer. Cover the pot and cook until rice is just cooked through, about 50 to 55 minutes. Stir in the shrimp, lemon juice, and half the scallions. Cover the pot and cook another 5 to 6 minutes until the shrimp are pink and cooked through. Uncover the pot and cook for another few minutes until any extra water is evaporated.

Garnish jambalaya with reserved scallions before serving. Serve with hot sauce on the side, if desired.

NUTRITIONAL INFORMATION

One serving: Calories 480; Fat 10.5g (Sat 2.5g); Protein 30.8g; Carb 66g; Fiber 6.5g; Calcium 159mg; Iron 4mg; Sodium 1573mg; Folate 87mg

---

Shrimp and Grits

MAKES 4 SERVINGS

A quintessential Southern dish, shrimp and grits is the ultimate comfort food. Grits, which are made from coarsely ground corn, are cooked until they reach a creamy, porridge-like consistency and are topped with sautéed shrimp. If you're pressed for time, you can buy instant grits, which cook much faster. This dish provides plenty of protein, calcium, iron, folate, and zinc.

Grits

4 cups water or low-sodium chicken broth

1 cup enriched stone ground grits

3 ounces grated reduced-fat cheddar cheese (about 1 cup)

1 tablespoon unsalted butter

¾ teaspoon salt

Shrimp

¼ cup low-sodium chicken broth

1½ tablespoons fresh lemon juice

1 teaspoon enriched all-purpose flour

3 slices center cut bacon (nitrate free), chopped

2 cloves garlic, finely chopped

1 pound large shrimp, peeled and deveined

3 scallions, thinly sliced plus extra for garnish

2 tablespoons chopped parsley plus extra for garnish

1 teaspoon hot sauce (adjust to taste)

Salt and pepper, to taste

To make the grits, put the water (or broth) and grits in a large heavy-bottomed saucepan and bring to a boil. Reduce to a simmer and cook, stirring occasionally, until liquid is absorbed, about 20 to 25 minutes. Stir in the cheese, butter, and salt. Keep the grits warm while preparing the shrimp.

Mix the chicken broth, lemon juice, and flour together in a small bowl. Set aside. Cook the bacon in a large skillet over medium heat until crispy. Remove the bacon from the skillet and set aside. Add the garlic to the skillet and cook for 30 seconds until fragrant. Add the shrimp and season with salt and pepper to taste.

Cook, stirring occasionally, until shrimp just turn pink, about 2 minutes. Add the scallions, parsley, hot sauce, and chicken broth mixture (stir the mixture before adding it to the skillet). Cook for another few minutes until the shrimp are cooked through and the sauce is thickened slightly. Stir in the bacon. Adjust seasoning to taste.

To serve, place a serving of grits in a bowl and top with some shrimp and sauce. Garnish with scallions and parsley. Serve immediately.

NUTRITIONAL INFORMATION
One serving: Calories 374; Fat 10.7g (Sat 5.1g); Protein 25.8g; Carb 37.9g; Fiber 2.1g; Calcium 173mg; Iron 2mg; Sodium 942mg; Folate 129µg

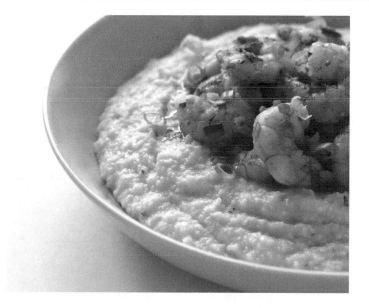

Seared Scallops with Creamy Corn

MAKES 4 SERVINGS

Many people think of scallops as gourmet, restaurant food but the truth is that they're very easy to make at home. Because they only take minutes to cook, they're perfect for busy weeknight meals. Scallops provide brain-boosting omega-3 fatty acids and are typically low in mercury. They're also a good source of lean protein; vitamin $B_{12;}$ and several minerals, including zinc.

2 tablespoons olive oil, divided
¼ cup minced shallots
2 cloves garlic, minced
4 cups fresh corn cut from the cobs
  (can use defrosted frozen corn)
¾ cup low-sodium chicken stock

2 ounces Neufchatel cheese
2 tablespoons chopped, fresh basil
  plus extra for garnish
1 pound large sea scallops (about
  12–16 scallops)
Salt and pepper, to taste

Heat 1 tablespoon oil in a large skillet over medium heat. Add the shallots and garlic and cook 2 to 3 minutes until softened. Add the corn and cook for another 4 to 5 minutes, stirring occasionally. Turn the heat up to high and add the stock. Cook for a few minutes until the liquid is reduced by half. Turn the heat off and stir in the cheese and basil. If the corn is dry, add a little more liquid until it is creamy. Season with salt and pepper.

Heat the remaining tablespoon of oil in a skillet over medium high heat. Pat the scallops dry with a paper towel and season them with salt and pepper. When the pan is really hot, add the scallops. Cook for 2 to 3 minutes without moving them until a golden crust forms. Carefully flip the scallops and cook for another 2 minutes on the second side until just cooked through. Serve scallops on a bed of creamy corn. Garnish with basil.

NUTRITIONAL INFORMATION
One serving: Calories 314; Fat 11.8g (Sat 3.5g); Protein 21g; Carb 34g; Fiber 3g; Calcium 36mg; Iron 1.5mg; Sodium 528mg; Folate 84µg

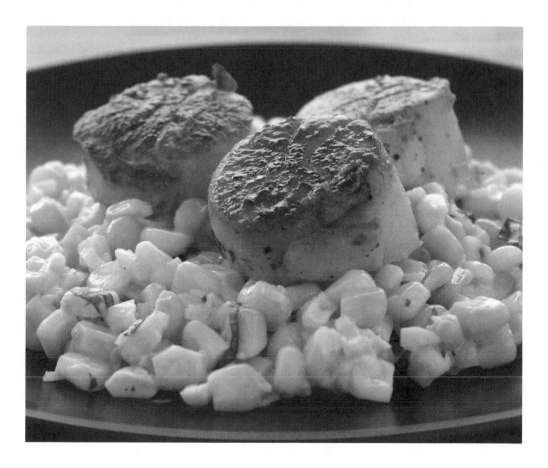

Mediterranean Shrimp Pasta

MAKES 4 SERVINGS

This colorful and nutritious pasta dish is packed with fresh seafood, artichoke hearts, spinach, and sundried tomatoes—all staples of a healthy Mediterranean diet. Artichoke hearts are a pregnancy super food and are packed with antioxidants and a wide variety of important nutrients. Save yourself a lot of prep time and buy them frozen. This dish has it all—omega–3s, protein, fiber, calcium, iron, zinc, Vitamin C, and folate.

- 8 ounces whole wheat angel-hair or thin spaghetti
- 1 tablespoons olive oil
- ¼ cup chopped shallots (about 1 medium)
- 3 cloves garlic, chopped
- ¼ teaspoon red pepper flakes (optional)
- 1 pound large shrimp, peeled and deveined
- 1 package (9 ounces) frozen artichoke hearts, thawed (can use canned)
- ½ cup sundried tomatoes, sliced
- 2 cups fresh spinach
- ½ cup reduced-sodium chicken broth
- 1 tablespoon lemon juice
- 1 tablespoon unsalted butter
- ¼ cup grated Parmigiano-Reggiano cheese
- Salt and pepper, to taste

Cook the pasta according to package directions. Meanwhile, heat the oil in a large sauté pan over medium heat. Add the shallots, garlic, and red pepper flakes and cook until softened, about 2 to 3 minutes. Add the shrimp and cook, stirring occasionally, until they just turn pink, about 3 minutes. Add the artichoke hearts, sundried tomatoes, spinach, chicken broth, and lemon juice and simmer for 2 to 3 minutes, stirring to wilt the spinach. Stir in the butter.

Add the cooked pasta and cheese to the pan and toss to combine all ingredients. Season with salt and pepper to taste.

NUTRITIONAL INFORMATION

One serving: Calories 442; Fat 10.6g (Sat 4g); Protein 29g; Carb 55g; Fiber 5.6g; Calcium 186mg; Iron 3.6mg; Sodium 892mg; Folate 360µg

---

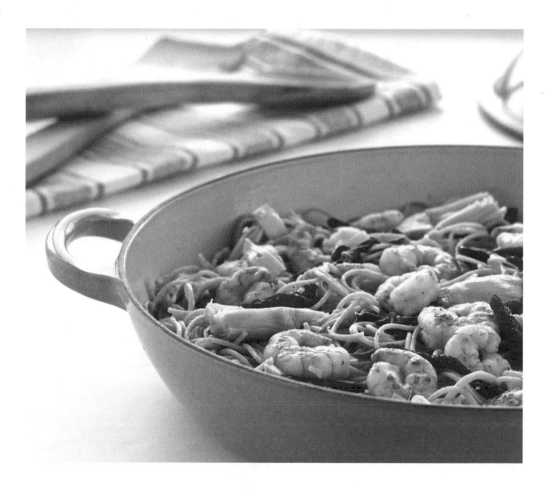

Salmon Oreganata

MAKES 4 SERVINGS

A simple topping of bread crumbs, herbs, lemon, and olive oil is the perfect way to dress up salmon for a quick weeknight meal. While it's cooking in the oven, make Sautéed Kale with Lemon and Garlic (page 222) to serve with it. Dinner in under 30 minutes and it provides plenty of healthy omega-3s to fuel the development of your baby's brain and eyes. How can you beat that?

½ cup whole wheat *panko* bread crumbs
1 clove garlic, minced
1½ tablespoons chopped parsley
¾ teaspoon dried oregano
Zest of 1 lemon

¼ teaspoon salt
1 tablespoon olive oil
4 salmon fillets (6 ounces each)
Lemon wedges for serving
Salt and pepper, to taste

Preheat oven to 400°F. Mix the bread crumbs, garlic, parsley, oregano, lemon zest, salt, and olive oil together in a bowl.

Place the salmon fillets on a greased baking sheet or in an oven-safe skillet (cast-iron works well). Season them with salt and pepper. Spoon the topping evenly over the salmon. Bake in the oven for 10 to 12 minutes, or until salmon is cooked through. Squeeze a generous amount of lemon juice on top before serving.

NUTRITIONAL INFORMATION
One serving: Calories 303; Fat 13.1g (Sat 2.1g); Protein 34.6g; Carb 6.6g; Fiber 1g; Calcium 53mg; Iron 2.2mg; Sodium 234mg; Folate 67mg

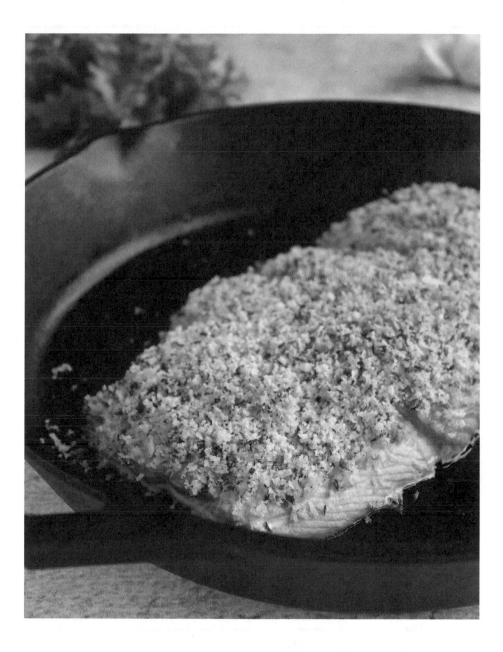

Caribbean Fish Tacos

MAKES 4 SERVINGS

These nutritious tacos have Caribbean flair! Pieces of fresh, grilled fish are enveloped in warm tortillas and topped with sweet mango chutney, creamy sour cream, and crunchy cabbage. These tasty tacos will provide you with plenty of omega-3s to help fuel the development of your baby's brain. You'll also get a good amount of protein, fiber, calcium, iron, and folate.

4 halibut fillets (about 5 ounces each) or other firm white fish like tilapia or cod
1 teaspoon dried thyme
1 teaspoon paprika
1 teaspoon onion powder
¼ teaspoon cayenne pepper
3 cups coleslaw mix (6 ounces)
1 tablespoon lime juice
4 teaspoons olive oil, divided use

8 small corn tortillas
½ cup mango chutney such as Major Grey's
½ cup reduced-fat sour cream or Greek yogurt
¼ cup cilantro leaves
Kosher salt and black pepper, to taste
Lime wedges for garnish

Cut the fish fillets into 1-inch wide strips and place them in a bowl. Mix the thyme, paprika, onion powder, cayenne, ½ teaspoon salt, and ¼ teaspoon black pepper together in a small bowl. Sprinkle the spice rub onto the fish and toss the fish to coat all of the pieces evenly.

Place the slaw in a large bowl and add the lime juice and 2 teaspoons oil. Toss to combine. Season the mixture with salt and pepper.

Heat a grill pan or skillet over medium high heat and brush the pan with the remaining 2 teaspoons oil. Add the fish to the pan and cook 3 minutes. Turn the fish over and cook another 2 to 3 minutes until opaque. Remove the fish from the grill.

Heat the tortillas according to package directions in the microwave or a skillet. Spread approximately 1 tablespoon mango chutney along the middle of each tortilla and top with about 1 tablespoon sour cream and a couple of pieces of fish. Top the fish with a small mound of the slaw and a few cilantro leaves. Serve tacos with lime wedges on the side. Squeeze some lime juice on top just before eating.

NUTRITIONAL INFORMATION
One serving: Calories 399; Fat 10.8g (Sat 3.6g); Protein 20.6g; Carb 4.7g; Fiber 1.1g; Calcium 81mg; Iron 2.5mg; Sodium 534mg; Folate 36mg

Black Cod with Romesco Sauce

MAKES 4 SERVINGS

A classic Spanish dish, Romesco sauce is one of my favorite no-cook sauces. It's made by pureeing heart-healthy almonds and olive oil with tomatoes, roasted red peppers, vinegar, and seasonings. This versatile sauce has a lovely red hue and bright, smoky flavor that complements grilled fish, chicken, or vegetables. Black cod, also known as sablefish, is one of the most concentrated food sources of omega-3 fatty acids. This dish is also rich in protein, B vitamins, Vitamin C, and plenty of minerals including iron.

½ tablespoon olive oil
4 black cod fillets (about 5 ounces each) or other firm white fish like halibut, tilapia or cod, skin removed
Salt and pepper, to taste

Romesco Sauce
4.5 ounces (¾ cup) jarred roasted red peppers, drained
½ small tomato, roughly chopped
2 tablespoons slivered almonds
1 large clove garlic
2 teaspoons Spanish sherry vinegar
1½ tablespoons extra virgin olive oil
¼ teaspoon smoked Spanish paprika
½ ounce bread, crust cut off
Salt and pepper, to taste

To make the Romesco sauce, place all of the sauce ingredients in a blender and blend until smooth. Season with salt and pepper to taste.

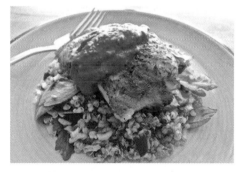

Heat the oil in a large skillet over medium high heat. When the oil is hot, season the fish fillets with salt and pepper and add them to the pan. Cook for 3 to 4 minutes until golden brown, then carefully flip and cook for another 3 to 4 minutes until cooked through.

Serve fish with a dollop of Romesco sauce on top. Serve extra sauce on the side.

NUTRITIONAL INFORMATION
One serving: Calories 379; Fat 27.8g (Sat 5.7g); Protein 20.6g; Carb 4.7g; Fiber 1.1g; Calcium 81mg; Iron 2.5mg; Sodium 534mg; Folate 36mg

Crispy Chicken with Tomato Arugula Salad

MAKES 4 SERVINGS

This lovely dish elevates the ordinary chicken cutlet by topping it with a colorful and vibrant tomato arugula salad. Arugula is a leafy green with a peppery flavor and a long list of nutritious compounds. This dish is rich in protein, calcium, iron, folate, and Vitamin C. Serve it right away so that the chicken stays hot and crispy.

Tomato Arugula Salad

4 cups baby arugula

2 medium ripe tomatoes, chopped

2 tablespoons chopped shallot (can substitute red onion)

2 tablespoons chopped, fresh basil

2 teaspoons olive oil

2 teaspoons balsamic vinegar

Salt and pepper, to taste

Crispy Chicken

¼ cup flour

1 egg

1 egg white

½ cup seasoned whole wheat bread crumbs

½ cup *panko* bread crumbs

4 (5 ounces) boneless skinless chicken breasts, pounded to ½-inch thickness

2 tablespoons olive oil

Salt and pepper, to taste

To make the tomato arugula salad, place the arugula, tomatoes, shallot, and basil together in a bowl. Add the oil and vinegar and toss to combine. Season the salad with salt and pepper.

Set up a breading station for the chicken. Place the flour in a dish. Whisk the egg and egg white together with 1 tablespoon water in a second dish. Mix the whole wheat and *panko* bread crumbs together in a third dish. Season the chicken on both sides with ½ teaspoon salt and ¼ teaspoon pepper. Working one at a time, dredge each breast first in the flour, then in the egg mixture and finally in the bread crumbs.

Heat the oil in a large skillet over medium heat. Place the chicken in the skillet and cook for about 4 minutes on each side, until the coating is golden brown and the chicken is cooked through. Remove the chicken from the pan and place on a serving plate. Top the chicken with some tomato arugula salad and serve any extra salad on the side. Serve immediately.

NUTRITIONAL INFORMATION
One serving: Calories 378; Fat 13.2g (Sat 2.7g); Protein 36.9g; Carb 22.8g; Fiber 2.1g; Calcium 82mg; Iron 2.3mg; Sodium 736mg; Folate 81g

---

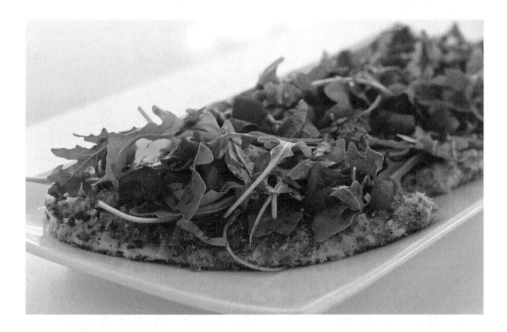

Slow Cooker Pulled Chicken

MAKES 10 SERVINGS

Slow cookers can be a busy girl's best friend. Simply toss all of the ingredients in when you head out for the day and when you get home, dinner is ready to serve. This pulled chicken is great to use in sandwiches, tacos, quesadillas, salads, pizza . . . you name it! It's rich in protein, iron, and B vitamins and also freezes really well, making it perfect for nights when you need a quick, nutritious meal on short notice.

1 small onion, finely chopped
3 cloves garlic, finely chopped
1 can (8 ounces) tomato sauce
¼ cup tomato paste
¼ cup cider vinegar
1 tablespoon Worcestershire sauce
2 tablespoons light brown sugar
2 tablespoons molasses
2 tablespoons paprika

2 tablespoons chili powder
¼ teaspoon cayenne pepper
1 teaspoon salt
½ teaspoon black pepper
1 pound boneless, skinless chicken
   thighs, trimmed of fat
1 pound boneless, skinless chicken
   breasts, trimmed of fat

Place all of the ingredients except the chicken in the bowl of a slow cooker. Add the chicken and turn to coat the pieces with the sauce.

Cover and cook on low heat for 6 hours. Remove the chicken and place it on a cutting board. Shred the meat with two forks.

Place the chicken in a large bowl and stir in enough sauce to coat all of the meat well. Save remaining sauce to serve on the side. Use pulled chicken to make sandwiches, tacos, and quesadillas, or to top salads.

NUTRITIONAL INFORMATION
One serving: Calories 154; Fat 2.7g (Sat 0.8g); Protein 19.7g; Carb 11.1g; Fiber 1.8g; Calcium 36mg; Iron 1.9mg; Sodium 379mg; Folate 11µg

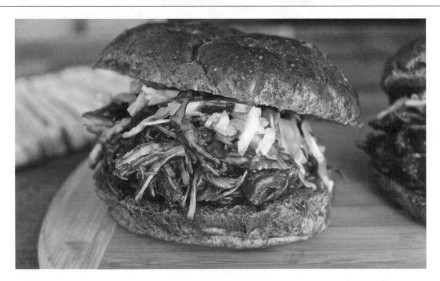

Spaghetti Bolognese

MAKES 8 SERVINGS

Spaghetti Bolognese is the ultimate comfort food. Who doesn't love a hearty bowl of slowly simmered meat sauce tossed with pasta and freshly grated cheese? This version, which uses turkey, is lighter in calories without sacrificing any of the rich flavor. This dish will provide you with plenty of protein and iron and by using whole grain pasta you'll get an extra dose of fiber as well. Milk is a traditional ingredient in Bolognese as it adds creaminess and tenderizes the meat. It also adds a boost of calcium.

2 tablespoons olive oil
1 medium onion, finely chopped
1 medium carrot, peeled and finely chopped
2 stalks celery, finely chopped
3 cloves garlic, finely chopped
¼ teaspoon red pepper flakes
1½ pounds lean (93/7) ground turkey
1 teaspoon salt, divided
¼ cup tomato paste
1 cup milk

1 can (28 ounces) crushed tomatoes
1 cup low-sodium chicken stock
1 tablespoon chopped, fresh thyme leaves
1 bay leaf
¼ teaspoon black pepper
1 pound whole wheat or multigrain spaghetti
Optional garnish: grated Parmigiano-Reggiano cheese, and chopped parsley

Heat the oil in a large, heavy pot over medium heat. Add the onion, carrot, celery, garlic, and pepper flakes and sauté until vegetables are softened but not browned. Add the turkey and season it with ½ teaspoon salt. Break the meat up with a wooden spoon as it cooks. Once it is browned, stir in the tomato paste and cook for another minute or two. Add the milk and simmer until it is completely reduced. Stir in the crushed tomatoes, chicken stock, thyme, bay leaf, ½ teaspoon salt and pepper.

Bring to a boil then reduce to a simmer over low heat. Simmer, uncovered, stirring occasionally to prevent the sauce from sticking to the bottom of the pan, at least 30 minutes until the sauce is thickened. Taste and adjust seasoning as desired. While the sauce is cooking, cook the spaghetti according to package directions. Drain the spaghetti, reserving about a cup of the pasta water. Add the spaghetti to the pot with the sauce and toss to combine. Add some of the reserved cooking water as needed to coat all of the pasta. Garnish with cheese and fresh parsley.

NUTRITIONAL INFORMATION
One serving: Calories 444; Fat 11.6g (Sat 3.2g); Protein 27.3g; Carb 56.4g; Fiber 4.9g; Calcium 118mg; Iron 4.8mg; Sodium 527mg; Folate 251μg

Chef's tip: To save time, chop all the vegetables and garlic together in a food processor.

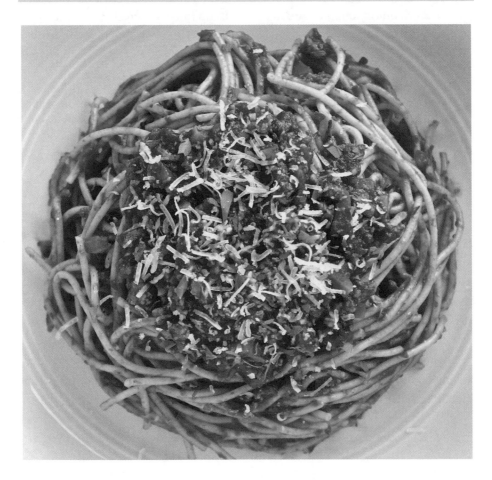

Pumpkin Turkey Chili

MAKES 6 SERVINGS

This hearty chili tastes like it's been cooked for hours but only takes about thirty minutes to prepare. The secret is the addition of canned pumpkin, chipotles in adobo and fire-roasted tomatoes, which give it plenty of smoky, slow-cooked flavor. Pumpkin adds a generous dose of Vitamin A, Vitamin C and fiber. This dish is also rich in protein, calcium, iron and folate. Chili freezes well so double the batch and store leftovers for after baby arrives.

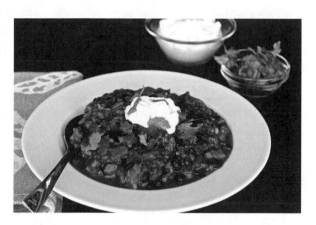

1 tablespoon olive oil
1 large yellow onion, diced
1 red bell pepper, diced
3 cloves garlic, minced
1 package (20 ounces) lean (93/7) ground turkey
1–2 chipotles in adobo, seeded and minced (depending on how spicy you like it)
2 teaspoons adobo sauce (from the can)
2 teaspoons ground cumin
1 teaspoon oregano
1 teaspoon salt

½ teaspoon black pepper
2 cans (15.5 ounces) black beans, drained and rinsed
1 can (15 ounces) canned pumpkin
1 can (14.5 ounces) diced, fire-roasted tomatoes
1 cup low-sodium chicken stock
3 tablespoons chopped cilantro
Optional garnishes: shredded reduced-fat cheddar cheese or reduced-fat Greek yogurt or sour cream, cilantro sprigs, chopped onion, and avocado

Heat the oil in a large Dutch oven or other heavy-bottomed pot over medium heat. Add the onion, pepper, and garlic and stir to coat with the oil. Cook, stirring occasionally until softened, about 4 to 5 minutes. Add the turkey and cook until browned, breaking it up as it cooks. Stir in the chipotles, adobo sauce, cumin, oregano, salt, and pepper. Add the beans, pumpkin, tomatoes, and chicken stock and stir to combine.

Simmer the chili, partially covered, about 20 minutes. Stir in the cilantro. Taste and adjust seasoning as desired. To serve, spoon chili into bowls and serve plain or topped with desired garnishes like cheese, yogurt/sour cream, cilantro, onion, and avocado.

NUTRITIONAL INFORMATION
One serving: Calories 369; Fat 10.4g (Sat 2.7g); Protein 30g; Carb 40.3g; Fiber 14.7g; Calcium 136mg; Iron 6.6mg; Sodium 845mg; Folate 127mg

Orecchiette with Kale and Turkey Sausage

MAKES 8 SERVINGS

My sister is a busy working mom who's always looking for fast and nutritious family-friendly recipes. This hearty pasta dish is one of her favorites. Kale is a nutritional powerhouse that works beautifully in this dish complemented by the sweet turkey sausage, bright lemon and nutty Pecorino Romano cheese. This meal is packed with plenty of nutrients including protein, fiber, calcium, iron, and folate. Orecchiette is a type of pasta that means "little ears" in Italian because of its unique shape. If you can't find it, you can substitute shells.

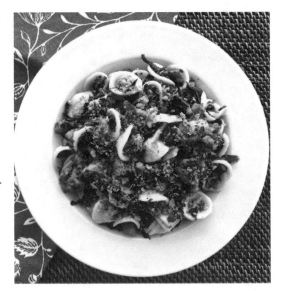

1 pound orecchiette pasta

2 tablespoons olive oil, divided

1 package sweet Italian turkey sausage (1.2 pounds), removed from casings

3 cloves garlic, minced

¼ teaspoon red pepper flakes

1 bunch Tuscan kale (about 1 pound), chopped

1 cup low-sodium chicken broth

2 tablespoons lemon juice

⅓ cup grated Pecorino Romano cheese (can substitute Parmigiano-Reggiano) plus extra for serving

Kosher salt and freshly ground black pepper, to taste

Bring a large pot filled with salted water to boil over high heat. Add the pasta and cook until al dente. Drain, reserving approximately 1 cup of the pasta water.

Heat ½ tablespoon olive oil in a large sauté pan over medium high heat. Add the sausage and cook until browned, breaking it up as it cooks. Remove sausage from the pan and set aside in a bowl. Drain any fat in the pan.

Add the remaining 1½ tablespoons oil to the pan. Add the garlic and red pepper flakes and cook until fragrant, about 1 minute. Add the kale and toss to coat with the oil. Sauté for 1 to 2 minutes, and then add the chicken broth and cover the pan. Cook until the kale is wilted, about 6 to 8 minutes. Add the lemon juice and season the kale with salt and pepper to taste.

Add the sausage, pasta, and Pecorino Romano cheese to the pan and toss to combine all ingredients well. Stir in the reserved pasta water, a small amount at a time until the pasta is just coated. Serve with extra cheese on the side.

NUTRITIONAL INFORMATION

One serving: Calories 398; Fat 10.2g (Sat 2.8g); Protein 24.3g; Carb 49.5g; Fiber 3g; Calcium 150mg; Iron 3.8mg; Sodium 503mg; Folate 242mg

---

Southwest Shepherd's Pie

MAKES 6 SERVINGS

Chef Gordon Ramsay has said that shepherd's pie is his ultimate comfort food. This version is packed with nutritious ingredients that provide a multitude of health benefits. It's rich in complex carbohydrates, protein, fiber, calcium, iron, potassium, folate, and a ton of other nutrients! The savory filling is flavored with smoky Southwest ingredients and it's topped off with a pillowy cloud of mashed sweet potatoes. So grab a bowl, curl up, and dig in!

Filling
- 1 tablespoon olive oil
- 1 medium yellow onion, chopped
- 1 red bell pepper, seeded and chopped
- 1 pound lean (93/7) ground turkey
- 3 cloves garlic, finely chopped
- 2 teaspoons chili powder
- 2 teaspoons ground cumin
- 1 tablespoon Worcestershire sauce
- 2 tablespoons tomato paste
- 2 tablespoons flour
- 1½ cups low-sodium chicken stock
- 12 ounces mixed frozen vegetables (like carrots, peas, corn, carrots, lima beans, and green beans)
- ¼ cup chopped cilantro plus extra for garnish
- Salt and pepper, to taste

Topping
- 2½ pounds sweet potatoes (about 3 large potatoes)
- ⅓ cup reduced-fat sour cream or Greek yogurt
- ½ cup low-sodium chicken stock, heated
- 1 tablespoon unsalted butter, melted
- Salt and pepper, to taste

Preheat oven to 400°F. To make the filling, heat the oil in a large skillet over medium heat. Add the onion and pepper and cook until slightly softened, about 6 to 7 minutes. Add the turkey and cook, breaking it up with a spoon, until it is no longer pink. Add the garlic, chili powder, cumin, Worcestershire sauce, and tomato paste and stir to combine. Stir in the flour and cook for another 1 to 2 minutes. Add the chicken stock and frozen vegetables and simmer another few minutes until thickened. Season with salt and pepper to taste. Pour the mixture into a 9-inch pie pan or 6 individual gratin dishes.

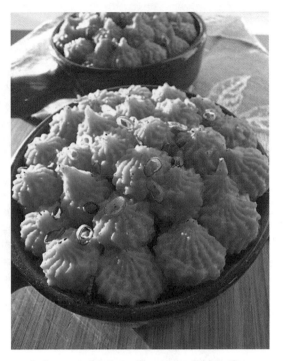

To make the topping, pierce the sweet potatoes all over with a fork. Place them on a plate and microwave for 8 to 10 minutes until soft, turning them over halfway through. Once cooled slightly, cut the potatoes in half and remove the skin. Place the flesh in a bowl along with the sour cream, chicken stock, and butter. Mash the mixture together with a potato masher until smooth. Alternatively, you can pass the sweet potatoes through a food mill or potato ricer and then stir in the other ingredients. Season the mixture with salt and pepper to taste.

Spread the sweet potato topping evenly over the filling, spreading it all the way to the edges. Alternatively, you can pipe the topping on with a pastry bag.

Place the pie(s) on a baking sheet and bake in the oven for 25 to 30 minutes until filling is warm and topping is lightly browned. Cool for 15 minutes before serving. Garnish with cilantro.

NUTRITIONAL INFORMATION
One Serving: Calories 420; Fat 12.5g (Sat 4.6g); Protein 22.8g; Carb 55.2g; Fiber 9.4g; Calcium 131mg; Iron 4mg; Sodium 265mg; Folate 63µg

Creamy Paprika Chicken with Egg Noodles

MAKES 4 SERVINGS

This comforting stick-to-your-ribs chicken and mushroom stew has Hungarian origins. Paprika infuses the creamy sauce with earthy flavor and gives it a lovely red hue. It's classically served over egg noodles but you can serve it with any type of pasta or even rice. This dish provides plenty of protein, fiber, iron, and several B vitamins, including folate and Vitamin B_{12}.

1½ tablespoons olive oil, divided
1 pound boneless, skinless chicken
    breast, cut into bite-sized pieces
½ teaspoon salt, divided
¼ teaspoon pepper, divided
1 tablespoon flour
1 tablespoon tomato paste
½ cup low-sodium chicken stock

1 small onion, finely chopped
2 cloves garlic, finely chopped
8 ounces cremini mushrooms, sliced
1 tablespoon paprika
¼ cup reduced-fat sour cream
8 ounces enriched egg noodles,
    cooked and drained
¼ cup chopped parsley

Heat 1 tablespoon oil in a large sauté pan over medium high heat. Season the chicken pieces with ¼ teaspoon salt and ⅛ teaspoon pepper and sprinkle them with flour. Toss to coat all of the pieces. Add the chicken to the pan in a single layer and cook without moving until golden, 3 to 4 minutes. Flip the pieces over and cook for another 2 to 3 minutes on the other side (the chicken will finish cooking later in the sauce). Remove from the pan.

Whisk the tomato paste and chicken stock together in a bowl. Set aside. Heat the remaining ½ tablespoon oil in the pan and add the onion. Cook for 2 to 3 minutes until it starts to soften and then add the garlic and mushrooms. Cook, stirring occasionally, until vegetables are tender, about 4 to 5 minutes. Add the chicken back to the pan along with the paprika and stir to combine well. Pour in the chicken stock mixture and season the sauce with the remaining ¼ teaspoon salt and ⅛ teaspoon pepper. Simmer for a few minutes until the sauce starts to thicken and the chicken is cooked through. Turn the heat off and stir in the sour cream.

Serve paprika chicken over egg noodles. Sprinkle with parsley before serving.

NUTRITIONAL INFORMATION
One serving: Calories 459; Fat 11.5g (Sat 3.4g); Protein 36.5g; Carb 49.2g; Fiber 3.7g; Calcium 65mg; Iron 4mg; Sodium 463mg; Folate 240µg

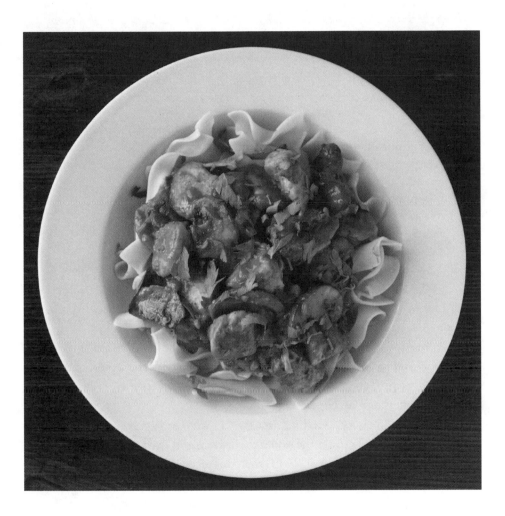

Balsamic, Maple, and Thyme Roasted Chicken

MAKES 6 SERVINGS

Amp up the flavor of everyday roast chicken with this dish that's nice enough for company but easy enough for a weeknight meal. Balsamic vinegar and maple syrup caramelize in the oven to give the chicken a crispy, golden brown skin, and fresh thyme adds a nice herbaceous note. This dish is packed with flavor as well as protein. Chicken skin can be enjoyed in moderation or to cut down on fat, remove the skin before serving.

1 lemon
2 tablespoons olive oil
2 tablespoons good quality balsamic vinegar
2 tablespoons pure maple syrup
2 tablespoons chopped, fresh thyme plus 5 sprigs

1 whole (4 pound) chicken, preferably organic
2 cloves garlic, peeled
1 teaspoon salt
½ teaspoon pepper

Preheat oven to 400°F.

Cut the lemon in half and squeeze 1 tablespoon juice into a bowl (reserve the other half of the lemon for the cavity). Mix in the oil, vinegar, maple syrup, and thyme.

Remove the giblets and any excess skin from the chicken. Rinse the chicken thoroughly and pat dry. Stuff the cavity of the chicken with the lemon half, thyme sprigs, and garlic. Lay the chicken breast side up in a cast-iron skillet (or other oven-safe skillet) or roasting pan.

Pour the maple syrup mixture over the chicken. Season the chicken all over with salt and pepper. Transfer the skillet to the oven and roast for 65 to 75 minutes, basting the chicken occasionally with the pan juices. Cook until an instant-read thermometer inserted into the deepest part of the thigh registers 170 to 175°F or when the thigh juices run clear when pierced with the tip of a small knife.

Remove the chicken to a cutting board or platter and allow it to rest for 10 minutes before carving. Skim and discard the fat from the pan juices. Carve the chicken and serve with the pan juices drizzled on top.

NUTRITIONAL INFORMATION
One serving: Calories 378; Fat 21.3g (Sat 5.9g); Protein 33.8g; Carb 6.9g; Fiber 0.2g; Calcium 31mg; Iron 2mg; Sodium 491mg; Folate 9μg

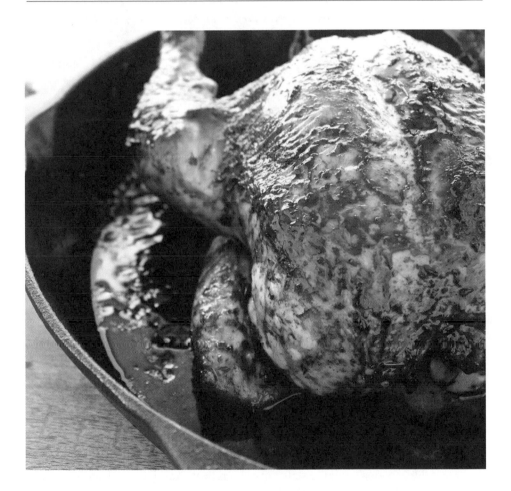

No More Takeout Beef with Broccoli

MAKES 4 SERVINGS

Put down the phone—you can make this delicious dish in the same amount of time it takes to get take-out. Beef is a rich source of protein and iron, which your body needs to produce red blood cells and fuel the growth of your baby and placenta. Broccoli is a pregnancy super food, supplying many important nutrients including fiber, Vitamin A, Vitamin K, folate, iron, calcium, and potassium. As an added bonus, it's also packed with Vitamin C, which will help your body absorb the iron in the beef.

1 pound flank steak, trimmed of fat
12 ounces broccoli florets (about 5 cups)
6 teaspoons safflower, peanut, or other high-heat, neutral-flavored oil, divided use

2 cloves garlic, minced
2 teaspoons minced ginger
¼ teaspoon red pepper flakes (optional)
Sliced scallions for garnish (optional)

Marinade
1 tablespoon low-sodium tamari or soy sauce

2 teaspoons cornstarch

Sauce
2 tablespoons oyster sauce
1 tablespoon low-sodium tamari or soy sauce

¼ cup low-sodium chicken broth
1 teaspoon cornstarch

Cut the steak in half lengthwise and then slice it crosswise (against the grain) into thin slices. Mix the marinade ingredients together in a bowl and add the beef to the marinade. Mix to coat all of the pieces. Let sit for 10 minutes.

Mix the sauce ingredients together in a bowl and set aside.

Meanwhile, heat, a large heavy skillet or wok over medium heat. Add the broccoli along with ¼ cup water and cover the pan. Let the broccoli steam for 3 to 4 minutes until crisp and tender. Remove the broccoli and place it in a bowl.

Heat 2 teaspoons oil in the skillet over high heat. Add half the beef in a single layer. Cook without stirring for a minute until browned then flip and cook another minute. Remove the beef and place in a bowl. Add another 2 teaspoons oil to the skillet and cook the remaining beef. Remove the beef from the skillet.

Heat the remaining 2 teaspoons oil in the skillet and add the garlic, ginger, and red pepper flakes. Cook, stirring often, for about 30 seconds. Add the beef and broccoli back to the skillet. Stir the sauce to mix it up and add it to the skillet. Cook, stirring constantly, for 2 to 3 minutes until the sauce is thickened and the ingredients are heated through. Garnish with scallions. Serve with brown rice or Quinoa Fried Rice (see page 232).

NUTRITIONAL INFORMATION
One serving: Calories 269; Fat 11.4g (Sat 2.9g); Protein 27.8g; Carb 10.1g; Fiber 2.4g; Calcium 74mg; Iron 2.7mg; Sodium 610mg; Folate 70µg

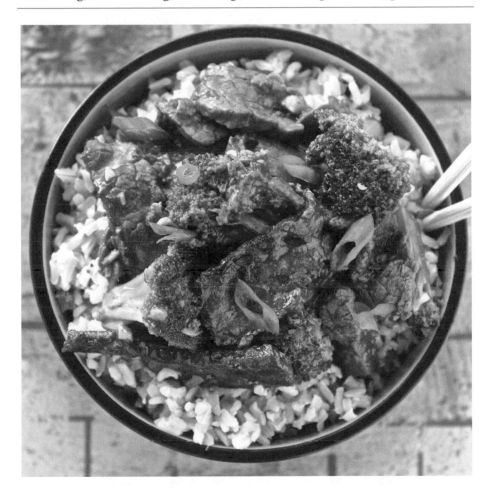

Grilled Skirt Steak with Chimichurri Sauce

MAKES 6 SERVINGS

Studies show that what you eat in pregnancy influences your baby's tastes, so experiment with bold flavors like the ones in this dish. Argentinian chimichurri sauce packs a punch with fresh herbs, garlic, and vinegar. It's commonly served with steak but it's also delicious with chicken, seafood, or vegetables. Skirt steak is a lean cut of beef and provides protein, iron, Vitamin B$_{12}$, and zinc. Be sure to slice it against the grain so that it's tender rather than chewy.

- 1 cup packed fresh parsley, roughly chopped
- 1 cup packed fresh cilantro, roughly chopped
- ¼ cup packed fresh oregano, roughly chopped
- 4 cloves garlic, chopped
- 1 shallot, chopped
- ¼–½ teaspoon red pepper flakes
- 1 teaspoon salt
- ¾ cup olive oil
- ½ cup red wine or sherry vinegar
- 1½ pounds skirt steak, trimmed of fat

Place all of the ingredients except the steak into the bowl of a food processor and pulse until blended but not completely pureed. Alternatively, you can finely chop all of the ingredients and mix them together in a bowl. Set aside about ¾ cup of the sauce in a bowl to serve with the steak. Season it with salt to taste.

Pour the remaining sauce into a large dish or resealable food storage bag. Cut the steak crosswise into three pieces and place them in the dish with the marinade. Cover and marinate in the refrigerator for 2 to 4 hours.

Heat a grill or grill pan to medium high heat. Remove the steak from the marinade and brush off the excess sauce. Place the steak on the grill and cook, without moving, until browned, about 4 to 5 minutes. Turn and cook another 4 to 5 minutes on the second side until done. Remove the steak to a cutting board and let it rest for 5 to 7 minutes. Slice thinly against the grain and serve with the reserved chimichurri sauce.

NUTRITIONAL INFORMATION
One serving: Calories 288; Fat 19.3g (Sat 5.1g); Protein 24.2g; Carb 1.5g; Fiber 0.5g; Calcium 30mg; Iron 3.2mg; Sodium 234mg; Folate 16µg

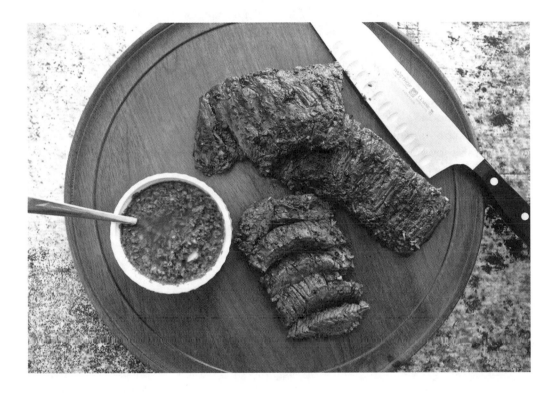

Sunday Beef Stew

MAKES 8 SERVINGS

This classic comfort dish is perfect for Sunday supper. Once all of the ingredients are seared in the pot, just throw it in the oven and in a few hours, you'll have a hearty meal that the whole family will love. Beef chuck roast is a lean cut of beef that gets deliciously tender after it's braised for hours. This dish is packed with protein, fiber, iron, and a full day's supply of zinc. It's also a good source of folate and calcium. Serve with Autumn Celery Root Puree (see page 230).

2½ pounds boneless beef chuck, trimmed of fat and cut into 1½-inch pieces
½ teaspoon salt
¼ teaspoon pepper
2 tablespoons olive oil, divided use
1 large yellow onion, chopped
4 cloves garlic, chopped
1 pound cremini mushrooms, large ones halved or quartered

2 tablespoons tomato paste
2 tablespoons flour
3 cups reduced-sodium beef stock
3 sprigs thyme
1 bay leaf
12 ounces baby rainbow carrots or 3 cups sliced carrots
2 cups frozen peeled pearl onions
¼ cup chopped parsley for garnish

Preheat oven to 325°F.

Season the beef with salt and pepper. Heat 1 tablespoon oil in a Dutch oven or large pot over medium-high heat. Add half of the beef to the hot oil and sear it on both sides until browned, 5-6 minutes. Transfer the meat to a plate. Repeat with the remaining oil and beef.

Add the onion, garlic, and mushrooms to the pot and cook a few minutes until softened. Stir in the tomato paste. Add the beef and its juices back to the pot along with the flour. Stir to combine well. Add the beef stock, thyme, and bay leaf, scraping up any brown bits from the bottom of the pot. Bring the mixture to a simmer and cover the pot. Transfer the pot to the oven.

Cook for 2 hours until the beef is just tender. Remove the pot from the oven and stir in the carrots and onions. Cover and return the pot to the oven for another hour until the vegetables are cooked through. Adjust seasoning with salt and pepper to taste. Garnish with parsley before serving.

NUTRITIONAL INFORMATION

One serving: Calories 291; Fat 10.2g (Sat 3.3g); Protein 34.5g; Carb 15.1g; Fiber 3.2g; Calcium 62mg; Iron 4.2mg; Sodium 373mg; Folate 40µg

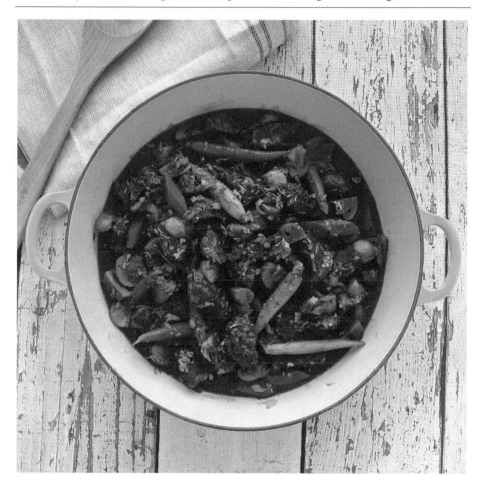

Rosemary and Lemon Grilled Lamb Chops

MAKES 4–6 SERVINGS

Lamb chops are paired with classic Mediterranean ingredients in this versatile dish that's elegant enough for a dinner party yet easy enough for a weeknight meal. Lamb is an excellent source of protein and Vitamin B_{12} and also supplies iron and zinc.

2 tablespoons olive oil
3 cloves garlic, minced
1 tablespoon chopped fresh
   rosemary
2 tablespoons fresh lemon juice

12 lamb chops (about 1½ inches
   thick), trimmed of any fat
Kosher salt and black pepper,
   to taste
Lemon wedges for garnish

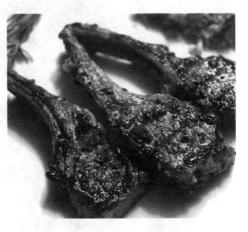

Mix the oil, garlic, rosemary, and lemon juice together in a large food storage bag. Add the lamb chops and seal the bag, turning the lamb to coat it with the marinade. Refrigerate for at least 1 hour or overnight.

Heat a grill or grill pan over medium high heat. Remove the lamb chops from the marinade and season them with salt and pepper. Grill the lamb for 3 to 4 minutes on each side, until cooked through.

Alternatively, you can broil the lamb chops. Preheat the broiler. Place the lamb chops on a baking sheet lined with foil or parchment. Broil 3 to 4 minutes on each side until cooked through. Serve lamb chops with lemon wedges on the side.

NUTRITIONAL INFORMATION
One lamb chop: Calories 256; Fat 12g (Sat 4.2g); Protein 31.5g; Carb 0.9g; Fiber 0.1g; Calcium 18mg; Iron 2.9mg; Sodium 75mg; Folate 1µg

---

Cheesy Quinoa and Bacon Casserole

MAKES 8 SERVINGS

This recipe was shared by my friend Lauren Kelly, the woman behind Lauren Kelly Nutrition (www.laurenkellynutrition.com). Besides being a nutritionist, recipe developer and food blogger, she's also the mom of three active kids and understands the importance of make-ahead-meals. The beauty of this casserole is that it can be prepared ahead of time and then baked off when you're ready to eat. And it only has five ingredients! This dish is rich in several important pregnancy nutrients including protein, calcium, and folate.

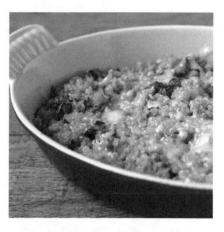

1½ cups quinoa, rinsed and drained
3 cups water
1 cup milk of choice
4 cups baby spinach

1½ cups shredded cheddar cheese
4 pieces of center cut, nitrate-free
   bacon, cooked and crumbled

Preheat oven to 350°F. Heat the quinoa and water in a large saucepan over high heat. Bring to a boil and reduce heat to low. Cover and simmer for 15 to 20 minutes until all liquid is gone.

Add the milk and spinach and stir until mixed well and spinach wilts. Remove from heat. Add 1 cup cheese and mix well. Transfer to a lightly greased 9 x 13 inch casserole dish and cover. Place in the refrigerator if you are baking later.

Bake in oven for 30 minutes until cheese is melted. Top the casserole with the remaining ½ cup cheese and crumbled bacon and broil for 4 to 5 minutes until lightly browned.

NUTRITIONAL INFORMATION

One serving (with reduced-fat milk): Calories 242; Fat 10.5g (Sat 5.6g); Protein 12.7g; Carb 22.8g; Fiber 2.6g; Calcium 221mg; Iron 2.1mg; Sodium 254mg; Folate 92µg

Cuban Mojo Pork Tenderloin

MAKES 4 SERVINGS

Pork tenderloin is a lean cut of pork that's a healthier alternative to higher fat cuts like bacon or pork chops. It's rich in protein, B vitamins, and minerals like zinc and selenium. This dish combines pork with classic Cuban flavors. The fresh citrus juice adds plenty of bright flavor as well as a hefty dose of Vitamin C. Serve this dish with Easy Black Beans and Rice (see page 234) or Maple Mashed Sweet Potatoes (see page 229).

1 (1 pound) pork tenderloin	1 teaspoon cumin
⅔ cup fresh orange juice	1 teaspoon dried oregano
⅓ cup fresh lime juice	½ teaspoon kosher salt
2 cloves garlic, finely chopped	¼ teaspoon red pepper flakes
2 tablespoons chopped cilantro	2 teaspoons olive oil

Trim any fat and silverskin (silver colored connective tissue) from the tenderloin. Mix the orange juice, lime juice, garlic, cilantro, cumin, oregano, salt, and red pepper flakes together in a bowl. Pour about half of the mixture into a one-gallon resealable plastic bag. Add the pork to the bag, close and refrigerate for at least 30 minutes or up to 4 hours.

Pour the remaining half of the mixture into a small saucepan and simmer on the stove for a few minutes until reduced by half. Reserve the sauce for serving.

When ready to cook, preheat the oven to 400°F. Heat the oil in a large oven-safe skillet over medium high heat. Remove the pork from the marinade (do not scrape off the solids) and add it to the pan. Cook for 2 to 3 minutes until browned on one side, then turn and cook for another 2 minutes on the other side. Place the skillet in the oven and cook for another 10 to 12 minutes, or until the internal temperature of the pork measures 145°F on a meat thermometer.

Alternatively, the tenderloin can be cooked on an outdoor grill. Remove the tenderloin from the oven and let it rest on a cutting board for 5 minutes. Cut into slices and drizzle the reserved sauce on top.

NUTRITIONAL INFORMATION
One serving: Calories 171; Fat 4.5g (Sat 1.1g); Protein 24.4g; Carb 7.1g; Fiber 0.5g; Calcium 27mg; Iron 1.8mg; Sodium 352mg; Folate 15µg

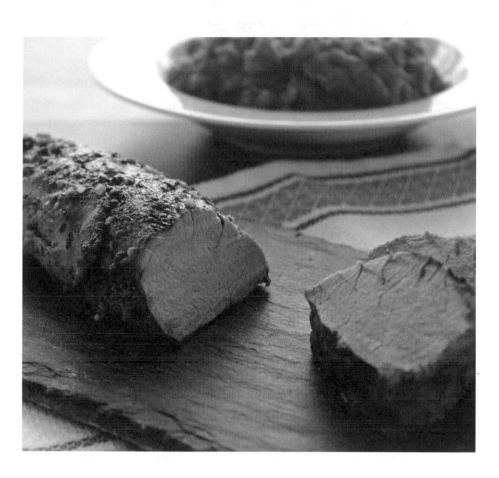

Spaghetti Squash Lasagna

MAKES 8 SERVINGS

This nutritious twist on lasagna uses spaghetti squash instead of pasta. Spaghetti squash has a mild, slightly sweet flavor and is packed with nutrients. The strands of squash are tossed with creamy ricotta cheese and chopped spinach. It's then layered with tomato sauce, mozzarella, and parmesan cheese and baked in the oven until it's bubbling with cheesy goodness. Packed with protein and fiber, this dish will keep you feeling full and satisfied. It also has a hefty amount of iron and folate and almost half your daily calcium needs!

1 large spaghetti squash (about 3½ pounds)

3 teaspoons olive oil, divided use

1 medium onion, chopped

3 cloves garlic, finely chopped

1 can (28 ounces) crushed tomatoes

2 teaspoons dried Italian seasoning

¼ teaspoon red pepper flakes

1½ teaspoons salt, divided

½ teaspoon pepper, divided

1 container (15 ounces) part skim ricotta cheese

1 large egg

5 ounces baby spinach, steamed and chopped (can use frozen spinach)

6 ounces (1½ cups) reduced-fat shredded mozzarella cheese, divided use

⅓ cup grated Parmigiano-Reggiano cheese

Chopped parsley for garnish (optional)

Preheat oven to 425°F. Cut the squash in half lengthwise and remove the seeds. Brush the flesh with 2 teaspoons oil. Place them cut side down on a baking sheet lined with parchment paper. Roast in the oven until tender, about 40 minutes. Remove from oven and cool. When the squash is cooled, scrape the flesh with a fork so that it forms spaghetti-like strands. You should have about 6 cups total.

Meanwhile, make the sauce by heating 2 teaspoons oil in a large sauté pan over medium heat. Add the onion and garlic and cook for 4 to 5 minutes until partially softened. Stir in the tomatoes, Italian seasoning, red pepper flakes, ½ teaspoon salt, and ¼ teaspoon pepper. Simmer the sauce for 15 to 20 minutes until thickened.

Meanwhile, mix the ricotta, egg, spinach, ½ cup mozzarella cheese, 1 teaspoon salt, and ¼ teaspoon pepper together in a large bowl. Squeeze all of the liquid from the spaghetti squash and add it to the bowl (the squash releases a lot of water as it cooks so make sure to squeeze it well). Stir to combine all of the ingredients.

Turn the heat on the oven down to 375°F. To assemble the casserole, spread about 1½ cups of the sauce on the bottom of an 8 x 11-inch baking dish. Add the squash mixture on top and spread it out evenly. Spread the remaining tomato sauce over the top of the squash and sprinkle the remaining 1 cup mozzarella and Parmigiano-Reggiano cheese on top. Bake in the oven for 35 to 40 minutes until bubbly and cheese is melted. Garnish with parsley. Let stand for 10 minutes before cutting and serving.

NUTRITIONAL INFORMATION
One serving: Calories 244; Fat 11g (Sat 6.1g); Protein 16.8g; Carb 21g; Fiber 4.4g; Calcium 448mg; Iron 2.8mg; Sodium 872mg; Folate 71mg

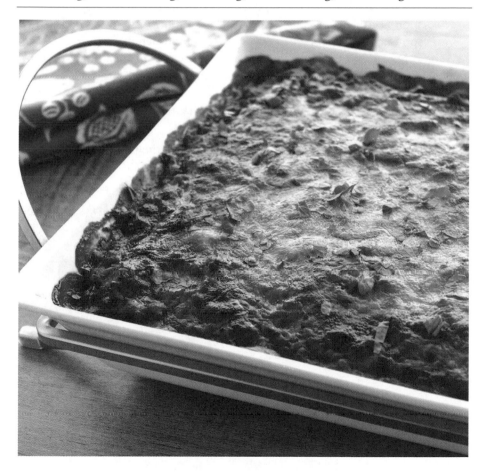

Chickpea and Spinach Curry

MAKES 4 SERVINGS

This dish was inspired by my mom who grew up in a vegetarian household. It's definitely a dish I turn to when I want something comforting that will deliver a taste of home. This vegetarian entrée has it all—protein, fiber, folate, iron and calcium, to name just a few! Serve it with brown rice, naan (Indian bread) or whole grain bread for a complete meal.

2 teaspoons olive oil
1 medium onion, finely chopped
2 teaspoons grated or minced ginger
1 teaspoon grated or minced garlic
½ teaspoon turmeric
¼ teaspoon cayenne pepper
2 cups chopped tomatoes (about 4 plum tomatoes)

¾ teaspoon kosher salt
1 cup light coconut milk
2 (15 ounce) cans low-sodium chickpeas, drained and rinsed
1 teaspoon garam masala
2 teaspoons lemon juice
1 package (5 ounces) baby spinach
Fresh cilantro for garnish

Heat the oil in a large sauté pan over medium heat and add the onion. Cook until softened, about 6 to 7 minutes. Add the ginger, garlic, turmeric, and cayenne and cook another minute until fragrant, stirring often. Add the tomatoes and salt and cook for another 5 to 6 minutes until the tomatoes break down. Mash them with the back of a spoon as they cook. Add the coconut milk and chickpeas and simmer a few minutes until the sauce thickens. Stir in the garam masala and lemon juice. Add the spinach and cover the pan for a few minutes until wilted. Uncover and stir the spinach into the sauce. Taste and adjust seasoning as desired. Garnish with fresh cilantro. Serve curry over brown rice or with bread.

NUTRITIONAL INFORMATION
One serving: Calories 291; Fat 9.1g (Sat 3.4g); Protein 12.1g; Carb 42g; Fiber 10.7g; Calcium 122mg; Iron 4.4mg; Sodium 702mg; Folate 230mg

Garam masala is an Indian blend of dried spices commonly used in Indian cooking. Most varieties contain a mixture of spices that includes peppercorns, cloves, cumin, coriander, and cardamom. It can be found in specialty grocery stores and increasingly in regular grocery stores. If you don't have it, you can use a little ground cumin and coriander.

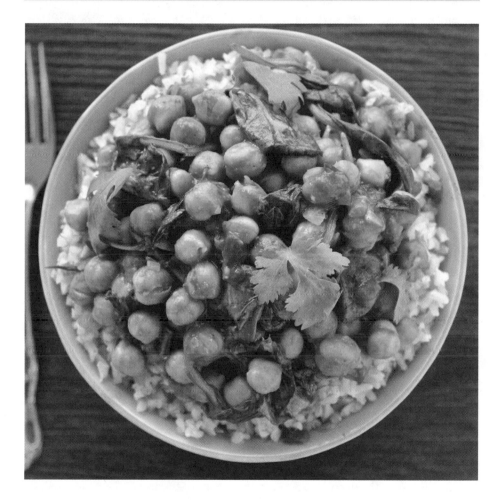

Roasted Sweet Potato and Black Bean Tacos

MAKES 12 TACOS OR 6 SERVINGS

These vegetarian tacos are hearty enough to satisfy even the biggest meat eaters! They're also packed with beneficial nutrients. Sweet potatoes and black beans are both terrific pregnancy foods and supply plenty of protein and fiber along with a host of important vitamins and minerals. Greek yogurt is the base of a cooling cilantro lime crema that's drizzled over the top. This dish is also rich in calcium, iron, and folate. Top them with Quick Pickled Shallots (page 123).

Roasted Sweet Potatoes

1½ pounds sweet potatoes (about 3 medium potatoes), peeled and diced into ½-inch pieces

1 tablespoon olive oil

1 teaspoon chili powder

½ teaspoon kosher salt

⅛–¼ teaspoon cayenne pepper (optional)

Black Beans

2 teaspoons olive oil

1 small yellow onion, chopped

2 cloves garlic, minced

2 (15 ounce) cans reduced-sodium black beans, drained and rinsed

1½ teaspoons chili powder

1 teaspoon ground cumin

½ teaspoon kosher salt

½ cup water

2 tablespoons chopped cilantro

Cilantro Lime Crema

½ cup nonfat or reduced-fat Greek yogurt

2 tablespoons chopped cilantro

1 tablespoon lime juice

12 small corn soft tacos, warmed

1 avocado, sliced

6 tablespoons crumbled pasteurized feta cheese

Cilantro leaves and Quick Pickled Shallots (see page 123) for serving

Preheat oven to 425°F. Toss the sweet potatoes with the oil, chili powder, salt, and cayenne. Roast in the oven for 25 to 30 minutes until tender.

Meanwhile, prepare the black beans. Heat the oil in a large skillet over medium heat. Add the onion and garlic and cook until softened, about 5 to 6 minute. Add the beans, chili powder, cumin, and salt and stir to combine. Add the water and simmer a couple of minutes until beans are heated through. Stir in the cilantro. Remove pan from the heat.

To make the cilantro lime crema, mix the yogurt, cilantro, and lime juice together in a small bowl.

To assemble the tacos, spoon equal portions of the black bean mixture and sweet potatoes onto each tortilla. Top with a slice of avocado, ½ tablespoon of crumbled feta, and some cilantro leaves. Serve with cilantro lime crema and Quick Pickled Shallots.

NUTRITIONAL INFORMATION
One serving: Calories 500; Fat 14.5g (Sat 3.2g); Protein 18.8g; Carb 80g; Fiber 20g; Calcium 160mg; Iron 5.7mg; Sodium 860mg; Folate 275mg

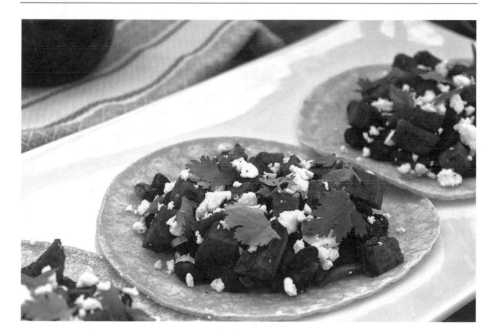

Pantry Pasta Puttanesca

MAKES 8 SERVINGS

This classic Italian dish is the perfect way to satisfy any salty food cravings! It uses nutritious, naturally briny ingredients like olives, capers, and anchovies and the best part is that they're all pantry ingredients that you can stock up on ahead of time. If you're not a fan of anchovies, don't worry. They add a nice salty flavor to the sauce and won't taste fishy. They're a good source of omega-3 fatty acids as well as protein, calcium, and iron.

2 tablespoons olive oil

4 cloves garlic, minced

2 teaspoons anchovy paste (leave out if vegetarian)

¼ teaspoon red pepper flakes

1 cup good quality black olives (like kalamata), sliced in half

3 tablespoons capers, drained

1 can (28 ounces) chunky style crushed tomatoes

¼ cup chopped parsley plus extra for garnish

1 pound cooked quinoa spaghetti or linguini (or other whole grain pasta)

Salt and pepper, to taste

Heat the oil in a large sauté pan over medium heat. Add the garlic, anchovy paste, and red pepper flakes and cook for 1 to 2 minutes until fragrant and anchovy paste is dissolved. Add the olives, capers, and tomatoes and cook, stirring occasionally, until sauce is thickened, about 10 minutes. Stir in the parsley. Season with salt and pepper to taste (the ingredients are salty, so you won't need much).

Add the cooked pasta to the sauce in the pan and toss to combine. Garnish with parsley and serve.

NUTRITIONAL INFORMATION

One serving: Calories 296; Fat 6g (Sat 0.9g); Protein 9.6g; Carb 51g; Fiber 4.5g; Calcium 66mg; Iron 3.9mg; Sodium 432mg; Folate 237mg

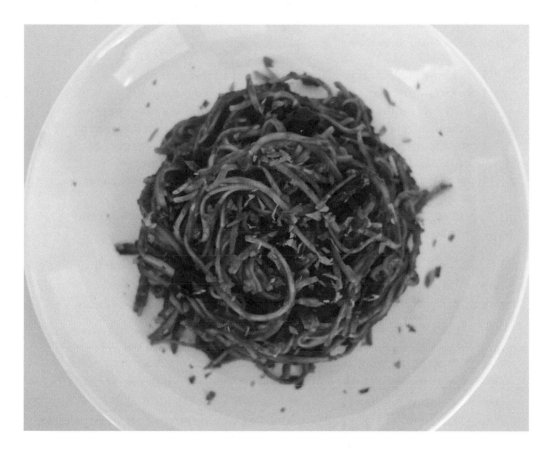

Thai Red Curry Tofu

MAKES 4 SERVINGS

Develop your baby's taste buds early with this flavorful Thai dish. Tofu is sautéed with a variety of fresh vegetables and fruit to provide a wide range of important nutrients. Tofu is a great source of lean protein, especially if you're vegetarian or vegan and are looking to boost your protein intake. This dish also provides plenty of Vitamin C as well as fiber, iron, and calcium. Serve it over brown rice for a helping of whole grains.

1 container (14 ounces) organic firm or extra-firm tofu

2 teaspoons safflower, peanut, or other neutral-flavored oil

3 tablespoons prepared Thai red curry paste

1 can (14 ounces) light coconut milk

1 tablespoon light brown sugar

1 medium red bell pepper, sliced into strips

2 cups snow peas

1 cup diced pineapple

1 tablespoon fish sauce or low-sodium soy sauce if vegetarian

2 teaspoons lime juice plus 1 teaspoon lime zest

¼ cup Thai basil or cilantro leaves

Salt, to taste

Brown or jasmine rice, for serving

Place the tofu on a plate lined with paper towels. Place another plate on top of the tofu and weigh it down with a couple of cans. This will drain the water. Let the tofu drain for at least 10 minutes while you prep the remaining ingredients. Cut the tofu into ¾-inch cubes.

Heat the oil in a large sauté pan over medium high heat. Add the tofu and cook, turning occasionally, until golden on all sides. Transfer the tofu to a plate.

Add the curry paste to the pan and cook for 30 seconds until fragrant. Add the coconut milk and sugar and stir to combine well. Bring the mixture to a boil then reduce to a simmer. Add the bell pepper and snow peas and cover the pan. Simmer for 5 to 6 minutes until vegetables are crisp tender. Uncover the pan and add the reserved tofu along with the pineapple, fish sauce (or soy sauce), lime juice, and zest. Simmer for another 3 to 4 minutes until ingredients are all heated through and sauce thickens slightly. Season with salt to taste. Stir in the basil or cilantro just before serving.

Serve curry over brown or jasmine rice.

NUTRITIONAL INFORMATION

One serving: Calories 220; Fat 11.8g (Sat 6.1g); Protein 10.8g; Carb 17.3g; Fiber 3.8g; Calcium 240mg; Iron 5.8mg; Sodium 623mg; Folate 53μg

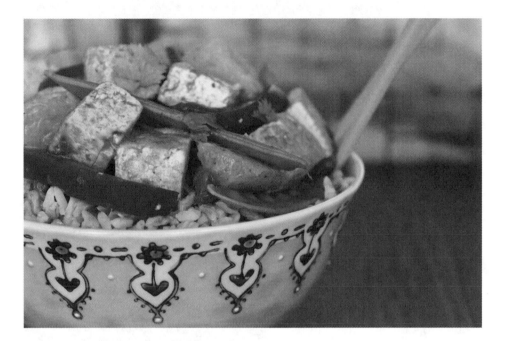

Lemon Risotto with Spring Vegetables

MAKES 6 SERVINGS

A staple in Italian restaurants, risotto is a classic rice dish that's not hard to make at home. The secret is in the stirring—adding the broth in stages and stirring frequently releases the starches in the rice, yielding a perfectly creamy texture. Vibrant spring vegetables and fresh lemon juice brighten up this dish and add plenty of nutrients. This dish is rich in protein, fiber, calcium, iron, and folate.

12 ounces asparagus
1 cup fresh or frozen spring peas
1 quart vegetable stock
1 tablespoon olive oil
1 medium leek, sliced (can substitute onion)
2 cloves garlic, minced
1½ cups Arborio rice

1 tablespoon fresh lemon juice
2 teaspoons lemon zest
2 tablespoons fresh, chopped parsley plus extra for garnish
½ cup grated Parmigiano-Reggiano cheese
Salt and pepper, to taste

Trim the ends from the asparagus. Cut the remaining stalks into 1-inch pieces. Bring a medium pot of salted water to a boil and add the asparagus. Cook until crisp tender, about 3 to 4 minutes. If using fresh peas, add the peas along with the asparagus. If using frozen peas, add them during the last minute.

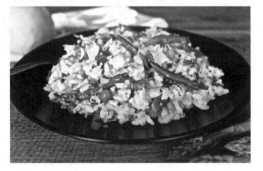

Transfer the vegetables to a bowl of ice water. Drain the vegetables and set aside.

Heat the stock along with 2 cups water in a large saucepan. Bring to a simmer and then keep warm on low heat while you make the risotto.

Heat the oil in a large, wide sauté pan. Add the leeks and garlic and season them with salt and pepper. Cook until leeks are partially softened, about 4 to 5 minutes. Add the rice and stir to coat all of the grains with the oil. Cook for 1 to 2 minutes to lightly toast the rice.

Add the warm stock, a few ladles at a time, stirring the rice frequently. Each time the liquid is almost completely absorbed, add some more stock. Continue adding the liquid in this manner, stirring often, to develop the starch in the rice. It should take about 20 minutes for the rice to cook. When the rice is done, it will be plump and al dente—tender but still firm to the bite. At this point, lower the heat and stir in the asparagus, peas, lemon juice, and zest, parsley and cheese. Season with salt and pepper to taste. Garnish with parsley. Serve immediately.

NUTRITIONAL INFORMATION

One serving: Calories 290; Fat 4.8g (Sat 1.9g); Protein 9.2g; Carb 50.2g; Fiber 4g; Calcium 125mg; Iron 4.2mg; Sodium 783mg; Folate 248μg

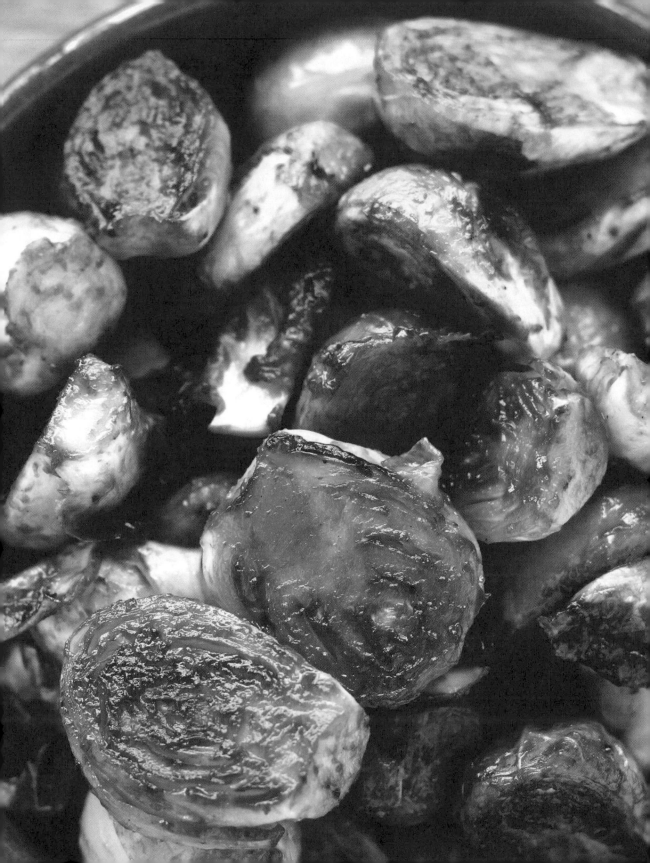

SIDE DISHES

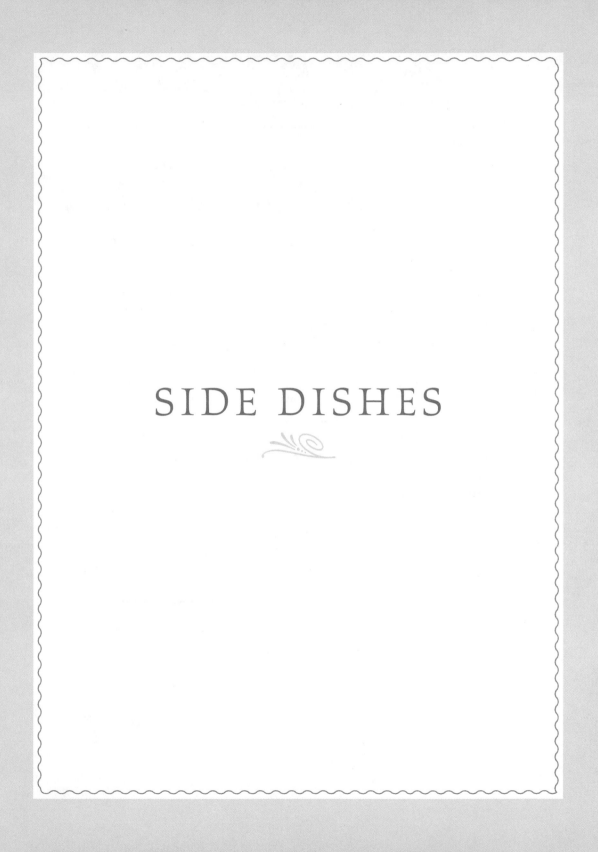

Miso Roasted Brussels Sprouts

MAKES 4 SERVINGS

These tasty little cabbages are coated with a salty sweet glaze and roasted in the oven until caramelized and tender. Brussels sprouts are packed with an abundance of vitamins, minerals, and disease-fighting antioxidants. This dish will supply you with a good amount of protein, fiber, and folate as well as a full day's supply of Vitamin C. Not sure what to do with any extra miso paste? Make Quick and Easy Miso Glazed Salmon (page 168).

1 pound Brussels sprouts
1½ tablespoons olive oil
2½ tablespoons white (shiro) miso paste
1 tablespoon maple syrup

1 tablespoon cider vinegar
1 teaspoon low-sodium tamari or soy sauce
½ teaspoon Sriracha or other hot sauce (optional)

Preheat the oven to 400°F. Cut off the brown ends of the Brussels sprouts and pull off any yellow outer leaves. Cut them in half lengthwise. Mix the oil, miso paste, maple syrup, vinegar, tamari, and Sriracha together in a large bowl. Remove about 1 tablespoon of the sauce and save it to toss with the Brussels sprouts later. Add the Brussels sprouts to the bowl and toss to coat them with the sauce. Transfer the Brussels sprouts to a baking sheet sprayed with olive oil cooking spray and spread them out in a single layer.

Roast Brussels sprouts in the oven until caramelized and tender, about 20 to 25 minutes. Stir them once or twice during cooking. Remove the tray from the oven and drizzle the reserved sauce on top. Toss to combine. Serve warm.

NUTRITIONAL INFORMATION
One serving: Calories 129; Fat 5.8g (Sat 0.9g); Protein 5.2g; Carb 16.6g; Fiber 4.9g; Calcium 58mg; Iron 1.9mg; Sodium 485mg; Folate 71mg

Braised Swiss Chard with White Beans

MAKES 4 SERVINGS

Looking to try a different leafy green? Swiss chard is a nutritional powerhouse in its own right. This veggie has an earthy flavor and is packed with a wide variety of vitamins, minerals, and fiber. The stems are also edible so if you like, you can slice them up and sauté them along with the shallots and garlic. This dish is rich in protein, fiber, calcium, iron, and folate.

1 tablespoon olive oil
¼ cup sliced shallots or onion
3 cloves garlic, thinly sliced
¼–½ teaspoon red pepper flakes
¾ pound Swiss chard leaves, washed thoroughly and chopped
1 can (15.5 ounces) cannellini (white kidney) beans, drained and rinsed

1 tablespoon tomato paste
½ cup low-sodium chicken or vegetable broth
½ teaspoon dried rosemary or thyme
2 teaspoons white wine vinegar
Salt and pepper, to taste

Heat the oil in a large skillet over medium heat. Add the shallot, garlic, and red pepper flakes and cook for 2 to 3 minutes until softened. Add the chard and cook, stirring often, until the leaves start to wilt. Stir in the beans, tomato paste, broth, and rosemary. Bring the mixture to a simmer. Cook until the chard is tender and the broth is thickened slightly, about 6 to 8 minutes. Stir in the vinegar. Season with salt and pepper to taste.

NUTRITIONAL INFORMATION
One serving: Calories 186; Fat 3.9g (Sat 0.7g); Protein 10.5g; Carb 29.5g; Fiber 6.8g; Calcium 132mg; Iron 5.2mg; Sodium 490mg; Folate 84mg

Sautéed Kale with Lemon and Garlic

MAKES 4 SERVINGS

This simple side dish is the perfect accompaniment to many of the entrees in this book like Salmon Oreganata (page 178). One can argue that kale is king among dark, leafy green vegetables. It's a nutritional powerhouse packed with fiber, antioxidants, vitamins, and minerals like calcium and iron. It's easy to cook and tastes great sautéed with garlic and a splash of lemon juice. The lemon juice also has Vitamin C, which will help your body absorb the iron in the kale.

1 tablespoon olive oil
2 cloves garlic, finely chopped
10 ounces chopped kale leaves
¼ cup low-sodium chicken or

vegetable broth
1 tablespoon lemon juice
Salt and pepper, to taste

Heat the oil in a large sauté pan over medium high heat. Add the garlic and cook about 30 seconds until fragrant (be careful not to let it burn). Add the kale and cook 1 to 2 minutes, stirring to coat the leaves with the oil. Add the broth and cover the pan. Cook 4 to 5 minutes until leaves are wilted. Uncover and add the lemon juice. Season the kale with salt and pepper to taste.

NUTRITIONAL INFORMATION
One serving: Calories 77; Fat 3.8g (Sat 0.6g); Protein 3.2g; Carb 9.5g; Fiber 1.7g; Calcium 117mg; Iron 1.5mg; Sodium 41mg; Folate 25mg

Sesame Roasted Broccoli

MAKES 4 SERVINGS

This is broccoli that anyone would love. When it's roasted at high heat, broccoli gets nicely browned and crispy around the edges. It's then tossed with a simple combination of Asian ingredients to enhance its flavor. This dish provides several important nutrients including fiber, protein, folate, and more than a full day's supply of Vitamin C.

1½ tablespoons sesame oil
1 teaspoon grated or finely chopped garlic
1 pound broccoli spears (florets plus part of the stems)

2 teaspoons sesame seeds
2 teaspoons low-sodium soy sauce
1½ teaspoons rice vinegar
Salt and pepper, to taste

Preheat oven to 450°F. Mix the oil and garlic together in a large bowl. Add the broccoli spears and toss to coat with the oil mixture. Transfer the broccoli to a baking sheet, spreading it out in a single layer. Roast in the oven, turning once, until the broccoli starts to brown, about 12 minutes. Sprinkle the sesame seeds on top and roast for another 5 minutes until the broccoli is cooked and sesame seeds are toasted.

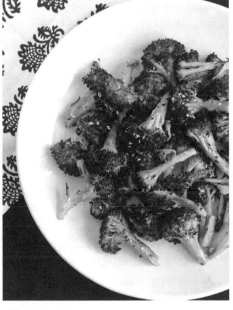

Remove the pan from the oven and place the broccoli in a bowl. Drizzle the soy sauce and vinegar on top and toss to combine. Season with salt and pepper to taste.

NUTRITIONAL INFORMATION

One serving: Calories 109; Fat 7.3g (Sat 1.1g); Protein 3.7g; Carb 8.4g; Fiber 3.2g; Calcium 69mg; Iron 1.1mg; Sodium 125mg; Folate 72mg

Oven-Roasted Vegetables

MAKES 6 SERVINGS

These colorful vegetables are packed with antioxidants, vitamins, minerals, and fiber. They're incredibly versatile too. Serve them as a side dish or use them in salads, sandwiches, pasta dishes, and frittatas. The garlic will soften and caramelize in the oven, leaving it with a mellow, sweet flavor. Use this recipe to make Roasted Vegetable Hummus Wraps (see page 124).

1 large red onion, peeled
2 bell peppers (yellow, red, or orange)
2 medium zucchini
4 carrots, peeled
12 whole cloves garlic, peeled
2 tablespoons olive oil
Salt and pepper, to taste

Preheat oven to 425°F. Cut the onion and peppers into 1-inch pieces. Slice the zucchini and carrots on a diagonal into slices that are roughly the same size. Divide the vegetables and garlic cloves between two baking trays lined with parchment paper. Spread them out in a single layer; don't overcrowd the pans. Toss the vegetables with oil and season them with salt and pepper.

Roast in the upper third of the oven until browned and tender, about 35 to 40 minutes, stirring them halfway through.

> **Note:** If using two shelves in the oven, rotate the pans halfway through cooking time to ensure even browning.

NUTRITIONAL INFORMATION

One serving: Calories 98; Fat 4.7g (Sat 0.7g); Protein 2.2g; Carb 12.6g; Fiber 3.2g; Calcium 42mg; Iron 0.7mg; Sodium 36mg; Folate 46mg

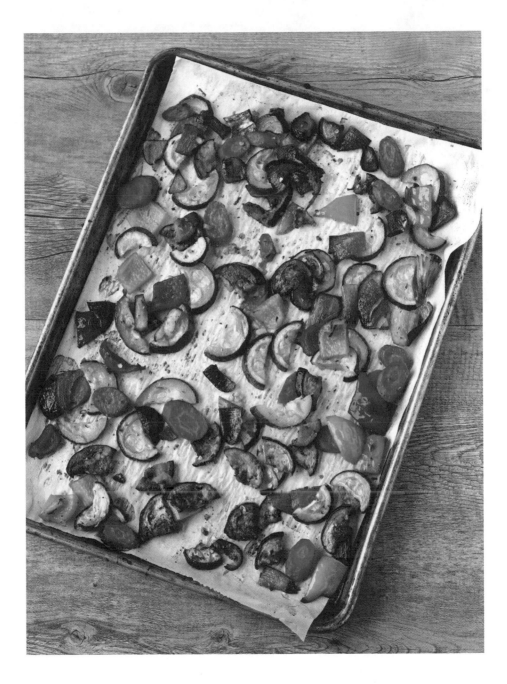

Sweet Potato Fries

MAKES 4 SERVINGS

There's no doubt that French fries are one of America's favorite foods but they're usually deep fried and loaded with unhealthy fats, sodium, and calories. Making your own fries at home is so much healthier, especially if you roast them in the oven and use sweet potatoes. Sweet potatoes have about the same amount of carbohydrates as white potatoes but they're full of antioxidants, vitamins, minerals, and fiber. Keep the skin on to retain more nutrients.

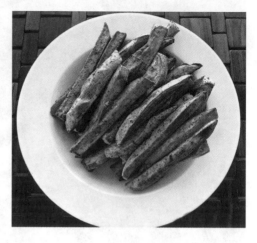

1½ pounds sweet potatoes (about 2 large potatoes), scrubbed and cut into batons (fry-shaped pieces)
1 tablespoon olive oil

1½ teaspoons chili powder
½ teaspoon kosher salt
¼ teaspoon black pepper

Preheat oven to 425°F. Toss the sweet potatoes, oil, and spices together in a large bowl. Arrange them on a baking sheet in a single layer. Roast potatoes in the oven for 15 minutes then flip them over and cook for another 8 to 10 minutes until cooked through. Serve warm.

NUTRITIONAL INFORMATION

One serving: Calories 179; Fat 3.5g (Sat 0.5g); Protein 2.8g; Carb 34.8g; Fiber 5.5g; Calcium 54mg; Iron 1.3mg; Sodium 400mg; Folate 18mg

Maple-Glazed Acorn Squash

MAKES 8 SERVINGS

A simple and elegant side dish, this acorn squash is just as suitable for your holiday table as it is for a casual weeknight meal. This sweet winter squash is often served stuffed but can also be sliced and baked for a quicker cooking time. As it cooks, the skin softens and becomes perfectly edible, so there's no need to peel it. Acorn squash is a good source of several nutrients including fiber, Vitamin A, Vitamin C, B Vitamins, and potassium.

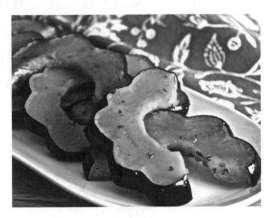

2 medium acorn squash
4 teaspoons olive oil
2 teaspoons chopped, fresh thyme

½ teaspoon kosher salt
¼ teaspoon black pepper
3 tablespoons pure maple syrup

Preheat oven to 400°F. Cut the squash in half lengthwise and scoop out the seeds. Slice the squash into ½-inch slices. Toss the slices with the oil, thyme, salt, and pepper. Arrange the slices on two lined baking sheets and bake for 15 minutes. Turn the slices over and brush with maple syrup. Bake for another 7 to 10 minutes until done. Serve warm.

NUTRITIONAL INFORMATION
One serving: Calories 82; Fat 2.3g (Sat 0.3g); Protein 0.9g; Carb 16.4g; Fiber 1.7g; Calcium 44mg; Iron 0.8mg; Sodium 149mg; Folate 18mg

Hasselback Sweet Potatoes with Sage and Parmesan Gremolata

MAKES 4 SERVINGS

These sassy sweet potatoes are a show-stopping side dish. Crispy on the outside with a soft interior, these potatoes are cut into thin slices and fanned out for a beautiful presentation. Sweet potatoes provide complex carbohydrates and fiber along with several important vitamins and minerals like Vitamin A, Vitamin C, B Vitamins, potassium, and manganese.

4 medium sweet potatoes, scrubbed
3 tablespoons olive oil, divided use
1 tablespoon chopped, fresh sage plus extra for garnish
1 tablespoon grated Parmigiano-

Reggiano cheese plus extra for garnish
1 clove garlic, minced
1½ teaspoons lemon zest
Salt and pepper, to taste

Preheat oven to 425°F. Place each sweet potato on a cutting board and line a chopstick up along either side. Carefully slice the potato into ⅛-inch slices, cutting almost all the way down to the bottom but not all the way through. The chopsticks will help prevent you from cutting all the way through the potato. Rub the potatoes with 2 tablespoons oil, coating the entire potato and getting down between some of the slices. Season them with salt and pepper. Place the potatoes on a baking sheet and roast in the oven for 40 minutes.

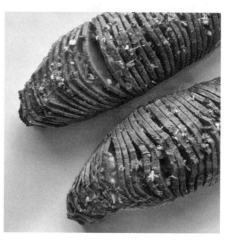

After 40 minutes, remove the potatoes from the oven and fan out the slices. Lower the oven temperature to 400°F. Mix the remaining tablespoon oil in a small bowl with the sage, cheese, garlic, and lemon zest. Spoon the mixture over the top of the potatoes and between the slices. Return the potatoes to the oven and cook for another 15 minutes until cooked through. Garnish with more sage and cheese before serving, if desired. Serve warm.

NUTRITIONAL INFORMATION
One serving: Calories 200; Fat 10.4g (Sat 1.7g); Protein 2.9g; Carb 24.3g; Fiber 4.1g; Calcium 67mg; Iron 1mg; Sodium 60mg; Folate 8mg

---

Maple Mashed Sweet Potatoes

MAKES 4 SERVINGS

You don't have to wait for the holidays to enjoy this easy puree. Creamy and sweet, you'll feel like you're diving into a decadent treat with this nutritious dish. Sweet potatoes are infused with maple syrup and cinnamon and topped with toasted pecans for a delightful crunch. This dish is packed with antioxidants, complex carbohydrates, fiber, and several vitamins and minerals.

1½ pounds sweet potatoes
1 tablespoon maple syrup
1 tablespoon unsalted butter
¼ cup low-fat milk

⅛ teaspoon cinnamon
⅛ teaspoon salt
¼ cup chopped pecans, toasted

Preheat oven to 400°F. Wash the sweet potatoes and pierce them several times with a fork. Place them on a lined baking sheet and roast in the oven until tender, about 45 to 55 minutes. Remove from oven and let the potatoes cool.

Put the maple syrup, butter, and milk in a large bowl and microwave until the butter melts and the mixture is warm. Scoop out the sweet potato flesh and add it to the bowl along with the cinnamon and salt. Mash all of the ingredients together with a potato masher, fork, or hand mixer. Adjust seasoning to taste. Transfer to a serving bowl and top with pecans.

NUTRITIONAL INFORMATION
One serving: Calories 221; Fat 7.7g (Sat 2.4g); Protein 3.6g; Carb 35.4g; Fiber 5g; Calcium 78mg; Iron 1.4mg; Sodium 127mg; Folate 12mg

---

Autumn Celery Root Puree

MAKES 4 SERVINGS

This healthy twist on mashed potatoes uses celery root as the main component. Celery root (also known as celeriac) is less starchy and lower in calories than potatoes and provides a good amount of Vitamin C, potassium, and fiber. Although it has an unusual, knobby appearance, it has a lovely, mild celery flavor and works wonderfully in purees. This dish has clean, bright flavors with a hint of tartness from the addition of a Granny Smith apple. Milk and a touch of butter add just the right amount of richness. It's the perfect side dish for my Sunday Beef Stew (see page 200) or at your holiday table.

1 medium celery root (about 1.25 pounds), peeled and cut into ½-inch pieces
1 small Idaho potato (about 6 ounces), peeled and cut into 1-inch pieces

1 Granny Smith apple, peeled, cored, and cut into 1-inch pieces
½ cup whole or 2% milk
1 tablespoon unsalted butter
1 bay leaf
Salt and pepper, to taste

Place the celery root and potatoes in a large pot of salted, cold water. Bring to a boil. Boil for 10 minutes and then add the apple. Continue to cook until tender, about 10 to 12 minutes.

Meanwhile, heat the milk, butter, and bay leaf in a small saucepan over medium heat.

Drain the cooked vegetables and return them to the hot, dry pot. Stir them over low heat for 2 minutes until dry. Pass the ingredients through a food mill or ricer into a large bowl. Gently stir in the hot milk mixture until smooth (remove the bay leaf). Alternatively, you can puree all of the ingredients together in a food processor. Season the puree with salt and black pepper to taste. Serve warm.

NUTRITIONAL INFORMATION
One serving: Calories 146; Fat 4g (Sat 2.5g); Protein 3.8g; Carb 25.4g; Fiber 3.3g; Calcium 96mg; Iron 1.4mg; Sodium 132mg; Folate 17mg

Roasted Asparagus and Grape Tomatoes with Balsamic and Pecorino

MAKES 4 SERVINGS

Bright green asparagus and vibrant red tomatoes come together in this side dish that's as flavorful as it is beautiful. Asparagus is chock full of powerful antioxidants, vitamins, and minerals including folate, which is crucial for preventing birth defects. It's also rich in protein and fiber. Additionally, asparagus has some natural diuretic properties and may help with leg swelling—talk about a pregnancy super food!

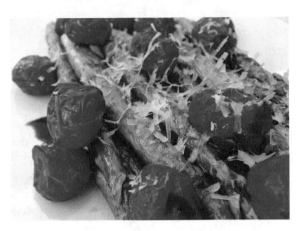

1 bunch asparagus spears, ends trimmed

1 pint grape tomatoes

4 teaspoons olive oil

2 tablespoons good quality balsamic vinegar

2 tablespoons grated Pecorino Romano or Parmigiano-Reggiano cheese

Kosher salt and black pepper, to taste

Preheat oven to 400°F. Place the asparagus and tomatoes on a baking sheet. Toss them with the olive oil and season with salt and pepper.

Roast in the oven for 15 to 20 minutes until the tomatoes are softened and the asparagus is crisp tender. Arrange the vegetables on a platter. Drizzle the vinegar on top and sprinkle with cheese.

NUTRITIONAL INFORMATION

One serving: Calories 93; Fat 5.3g (Sat 1.1g); Protein 4.2g; Carb 8.8g; Fiber 3.3g; Calcium 63mg; Iron 2.7mg; Sodium 45mg; Folate 70mg

Quinoa Fried "Rice"

MAKES 4 SERVINGS

Protein-packed quinoa replaces white rice in this classic Chinese dish. Quinoa is a gluten-free whole grain that provides a variety of vitamins, minerals, and fiber to boost the health benefits of this dish. Add some tofu, chicken, or shrimp and this fried "rice" easily becomes a main course. Cooled quinoa works best in this dish so plan ahead and use leftover quinoa from the night before. This recipe is rich in protein, fiber, iron, and B vitamins, including folate. Plus, the ginger may help alleviate nausea.

1 cup quinoa, rinsed
4 teaspoons safflower, peanut, or other neutral-flavored oil, divided
2 eggs
3 cloves garlic, minced
1 tablespoon minced ginger
3 scallions, sliced (whites and greens separated) plus extra for garnish

1 ¼ cups frozen peas and carrots, defrosted
2 tablespoons low-sodium soy sauce (or tamari if gluten-free)
2 teaspoons sesame oil
½ teaspoon Sriracha or other hot sauce (optional)
Salt and pepper, to taste

Place the quinoa in a saucepan with 2 cups water and bring to a boil. Lower heat to a simmer and cover. Cook for 10 to 15 minutes until done. Cool the quinoa, ideally overnight in the refrigerator.

Heat 1 teaspoon oil in a wok over medium high heat. Beat the eggs in a bowl with a fork and add them to the pan. Season them with a pinch of salt and pepper. Cook, stirring occasionally, until firm. Break the egg up with a spatula and transfer it to a plate.

Heat the remaining 3 teaspoons oil in the wok. Add the garlic, ginger, and scallion whites and cook until fragrant, about 2 to 3 minutes. Add the peas and carrots and cook until heated. Add the cooled quinoa and stir to combine. Add the soy sauce, sesame oil, Sriracha, scallion greens, and cooked egg and stir to combine well. Garnish with scallion greens.

NUTRITIONAL INFORMATION
One serving: Calories 283; Fat 10.9g (Sat 1.8g); Protein 11.1g; Carb 35.1g; Fiber 5g; Calcium 56mg; Iron 3.2mg; Sodium 348mg; Folate 109µg

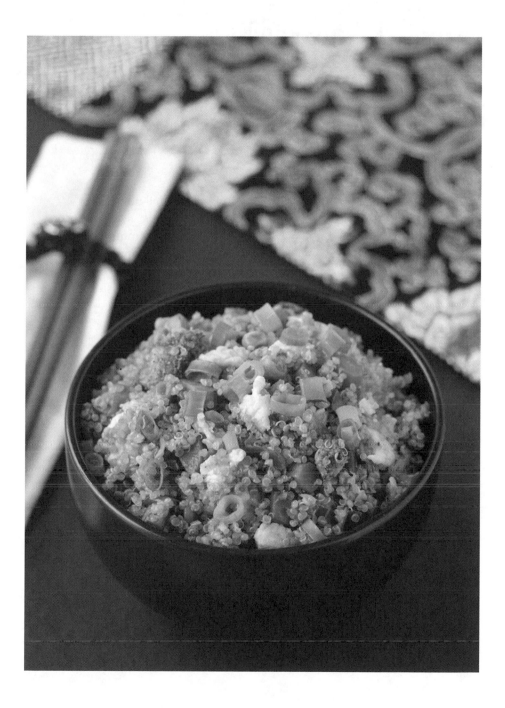

Easy Black Beans and Rice

MAKES 4 SERVINGS

This classic dish is a staple in many cultures. The combination of rice and beans provides all nine essential amino acids, making this dish a complete protein. In addition it's a great source of whole grains, fiber, and several other nutrients including iron, folate, and zinc. Using instant brown rice provides the same nutritional values as regular brown rice but cooks in a quarter of the time. Eating healthy just got a lot easier.

2 teaspoons olive oil
1 small onion, chopped
2 cloves garlic, chopped
2 cups instant brown rice
1¾ cups vegetable broth, chicken
   broth, or water

1 teaspoon chili powder
1 can (15.5 ounces) low-sodium
   black beans, drained and rinsed
2 tablespoons chopped cilantro
   (optional)
Salt and pepper, to taste

Heat the oil in a medium saucepan over medium heat. Add the onion and garlic and cook for a few minutes until softened. Stir in the rice, broth and chili powder. Bring the liquid to a boil then reduce to a simmer, cover, and cook for 5 minutes. Remove from heat and stir in the beans. Cover and let stand 5 more minutes. Season the rice and beans with salt and pepper to taste. Stir in the cilantro just before serving.

NUTRITIONAL INFORMATION
One serving: Calories 286; Fat 4.2g (Sat 0.3g); Protein 9.3g; Carb 57.2g; Fiber 7.6g; Calcium 38mg; Iron 2.9mg; Sodium 255mg; Folate 166μg

Mediterranean Quinoa

MAKES 4 SERVINGS

This super simple, nutritious side dish features quinoa, a powerful and versatile whole grain. You can use it in place of rice in most dishes and it cooks up a lot faster. Baby spinach and sun-dried tomatoes add nutrients and flavor to this Mediterranean-inspired dish, but feel free to stir in your favorite ingredients. This dish will provide you with a boost of protein, fiber, iron, and folate.

2 teaspoons olive oil
2 cloves garlic, minced
1 cup quinoa, rinsed
2 cups low-sodium chicken or
   vegetable broth

2 cups baby spinach, roughly torn
2 tablespoons chopped sundried
   tomatoes, drained
Salt and pepper, to taste

Heat the oil in a medium saucepan over medium heat. Add the garlic and cook for 1 to 2 minutes until fragrant. Add the quinoa and cook, stirring often, about 2 to 3 minutes, until toasted. Pour in the broth and bring to a boil. Reduce heat to a simmer, cover the pan, and cook for 10 to 15 minutes until quinoa is cooked.

Stir in the spinach and sundried tomatoes. Cover the pan and cook on low heat for a few minutes until the spinach is wilted. Season the quinoa with salt and pepper. Fluff with a fork before serving.

NUTRITIONAL INFORMATION
One serving: Calories 194; Fat 5.1g (Sat 0.7g); Protein 6.7g; Carb 30.6g; Fiber 3.5g; Calcium 38mg; Iron 2.5mg; Sodium 85mg; Folate 107µg

Savory Tomato Cobbler

MAKES 8 SERVINGS

This mouthwatering dish is from Melissa, the multitalented woman behind the blog ChinDeep (www.chindeep.com). On her site, Melissa writes about how to add simple pleasures to your life every day and this delicious cobbler would certainly do just that! This recipe tastes like summer. It features succulent tomatoes, which are topped with a basil-infused biscuit dough and baked until golden brown and bubbling. This dish provides protein, calcium, iron, and folate as well as plenty of Vitamin C.

5 large (or 10 small) tomatoes, chopped	¼ teaspoon baking soda
1 tablespoon cornstarch	4 tablespoons cold unsalted butter, cut into chunks
2 tablespoons sugar, divided	1 large egg, beaten
1 teaspoon sea salt	¾ cup reduced-fat buttermilk
1 teaspoon freshly ground pepper	¼ cup chopped, fresh basil
1 cup all-purpose flour	½ teaspoon onion powder
1 cup cornmeal	½ teaspoon garlic powder
1½ teaspoons baking powder	Salt, to taste

Preheat oven to 375°F. Butter a 10-inch, deep-dish, glass pie plate or a 9 × 9-inch square, glass baking dish. In a large bowl, toss the chopped tomatoes with the cornstarch, 1 tablespoon sugar, and the salt and pepper. Transfer the mixture to the baking dish.

In the bowl of a large food processor, combine the flour, cornmeal, baking powder, baking soda, reserved 1 tablespoon sugar, and butter. Season with salt to taste. Pulse until big crumbs form. Add the beaten egg and buttermilk. Pulse until the mixture forms a ball. If the dough seems too dry, and doesn't hold together, add more buttermilk, a tablespoonful at a time, until it does. If the dough seems too wet, add more flour, a tablespoonful at a time, until it forms a ball. Once you have the dough the right consistency, fold in the basil.

Drop the dough by tablespoons onto the tomatoes in the dish, leaving spaces between the dough so that steam can escape and the tomato mixture has a chance to thicken a bit. Sprinkle the top with the onion powder and garlic powder. Bake for 45 to 50 minutes, until crust is golden brown and tomatoes are bubbling underneath. Cool to room temperature and serve.

NUTRITIONAL INFORMATION

One serving: Calories 267; Fat 7g (Sat 4.3g); Protein 8.8g; Carb 41.5g; Fiber 2.7g; Calcium 206mg; Iron 2.2mg; Sodium 496mg; Folate 136µg

---

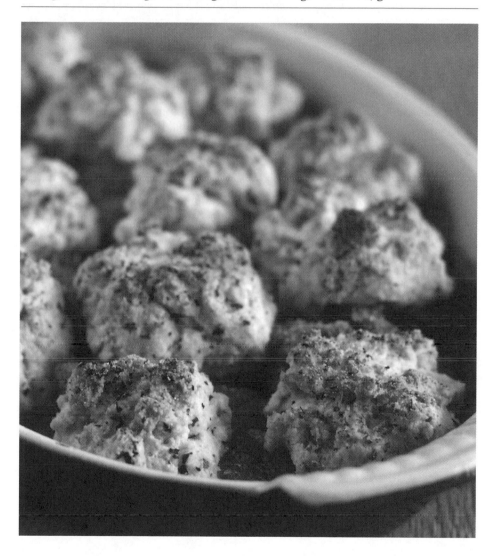

Preggo Parmesan and Herb Popovers

MAKES 12 POPOVERS

These lovely treats would be right at home at a spring lunch or an elegant dinner party. The perfect popover should be golden brown and crusty on the outside and light and airy on the inside. They get their height from the blast of high heat in a very hot oven so don't open the door to peek while they're baking! This dish will provide you with whole grains, protein and folate.

3 large eggs, at room temperature
1½ cups warm reduced-fat (2%) milk
¾ teaspoon kosher salt
1 cup all-purpose flour
½ cup white whole wheat flour

⅓ cup plus 1 tablespoon grated Parmesan cheese, divided use
3 tablespoons chopped, fresh herbs (like dill, basil, oregano, and thyme) plus extra for garnish

Preheat oven to 450°F. Whisk the eggs in a large bowl until light yellow and frothy. Add the milk and salt and whisk again until combined. Add both of the flours, all at once. Whisk just until a thin batter forms—do not over-mix. The batter may have small lumps. Gently whisk in ⅓ cup Parmesan cheese and herbs until just combined. Let the batter rest for 20 minutes while the oven heats up.

Heat a standard 12-cup muffin pan in the oven for a few minutes until hot. Remove the pan and spray generously with cooking spray. Pour the batter into the wells—they should be about ¾ full. Sprinkle ¼ teaspoon Parmesan on top of each one and garnish with fresh herbs.

Place the pan in the middle or lower third of the oven. Bake for 20 minutes until the popovers are puffed up and golden brown. Do not open the oven door while they bake. Reduce the temperature to 350°F and bake for another 12 to 15 minutes until done. Remove the popovers from the oven and cut slits in the tops with a sharp knife to prevent them from collapsing. Serve immediately.

NUTRITIONAL INFORMATION
One popover: Calories 102; Fat 2.7g (Sat 1.4g); Protein 5.6g; Carb 13.3g; Fiber 0.8g; Calcium 83mg; Iron 0.9mg; Sodium 228mg; Folate 40µg

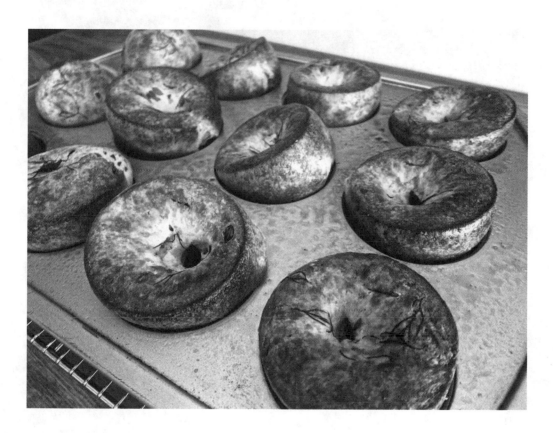

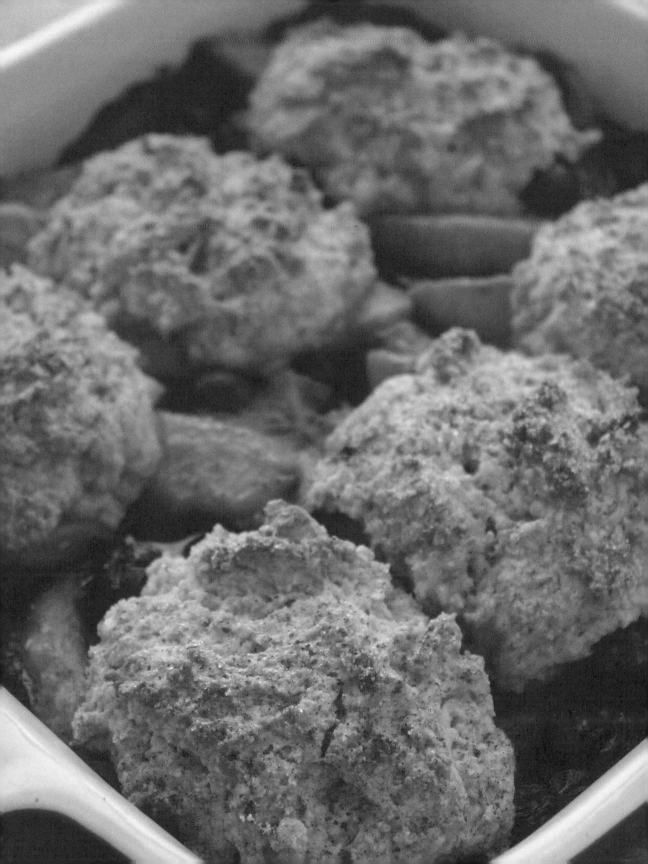

DESSERTS

Baby on Board Blueberry Peach Cobbler

MAKES 6 SERVINGS

For a tasty finale to any meal, try this cobbler that's brimming with summer fruit. Fresh juicy peaches and vibrant blueberries are baked beneath a layer of fluffy biscuits. Using white whole wheat flour in the biscuit dough adds a helping of nutritious whole grains. This dish supplies a good amount of antioxidants, fiber, Vitamin C, and folate. Serve the cobbler with ice cream or whipped cream.

Filling
- 4½ cups sliced, peeled peaches (4–5 medium peaches)
- 1½ cups blueberries
- 2–3 tablespoons sugar (depending on the sweetness of the fruit)
- 2 tablespoons flour
- ¼ teaspoon cinnamon
- 1 tablespoon lemon juice
- Zest of 1 lemon

Biscuit Topping
- 6 tablespoons all-purpose flour
- 6 tablespoons white whole wheat flour
- 1 teaspoon baking powder
- ¼ teaspoon baking soda
- ¼ teaspoon salt
- 2 tablespoons plus ½ teaspoon sugar, divided
- 3 tablespoons cold, unsalted butter, diced
- 6 tablespoons buttermilk
- ⅛ teaspoon cinnamon

Preheat oven to 400°F. Place the peaches and blueberries in a large bowl. Add the sugar, flour, cinnamon, lemon juice, and zest and toss to combine well. Transfer the mixture to a 9 x 9-inch square baking dish sprayed with cooking spray. Bake in the oven for 10 minutes. Remove from oven.

Meanwhile, make the biscuit topping. Whisk both types of flour, baking powder, baking soda, salt, and 2 tablespoons sugar together in a bowl. Add the butter and using a pastry cutter or your fingers, incorporate the butter in the dry ingredients until the mixture resembles a coarse meal. Add the buttermilk and stir until just moistened. Do not over-mix.

Drop the batter onto the fruit, forming six mounds. Sprinkle the remaining ½ teaspoon sugar and the cinnamon on top. Bake for 25 to 30 minutes, until the fruit is bubbly and the top is golden. Let stand for 10 minutes before serving.

NUTRITIONAL INFORMATION

One serving: Calories 239; Fat 6.2g (Sat 4g); Protein 5.7g; Carb 42.1g; Fiber 3.8g; Calcium 138mg; Iron 1.3mg; Sodium 264mg; Folate 42µg

---

Cannoli Cream-Filled Strawberries

MAKES ABOUT 24 STRAWBERRIES

These adorable treats were shared by my friend Justine over at Full Belly Sisters (www. fullbellysisters.blogspot.com). Justine takes the silky-smooth creamy filling that's traditionally used to stuff cannoli and gives it a new home—the strawberry. Strawberries are bursting with antioxidants, Vitamin C, and fiber and the cannoli cream adds a boost of protein and calcium. Serve these tasty morsels at your next party and watch as they quickly disappear.

24 strawberries, cleaned and dried
1¼ cup good quality ricotta cheese
2 ounces reduced-fat cream cheese
2 tablespoons powdered sugar
1–2 teaspoons honey
½ teaspoon vanilla
¼ teaspoon lemon zest
Shaved dark chocolate or lemon zest (for garnish)

Trim the top and bottoms of the strawberries, so that they are level and can stand. Cut or scoop out the tops of the berries. Put the ricotta, cream cheese, sugar, honey, vanilla, and lemon zest into a food processor. Process for 3 to 4 minutes, until the mixture is thick and smooth. Pipe or spoon the cannoli cream into the berries.

Garnish with shaved dark chocolate or lemon zest.

NUTRITIONAL INFORMATION

One strawberry: Calories 35; Fat 2.1g (Sat 1.4g); Protein 1.7g; Carb 2.3g; Fiber 0.2g; Calcium 31mg; Iron 0.1mg; Sodium 18mg; Folate 4mg

---

Mixed Berry Crumble

MAKES 8 SERVINGS

This dish is a guaranteed crowd pleaser! This lovely dessert is bursting with juicy, vibrant berries, which are packed with disease-fighting antioxidants, Vitamin C, and fiber. The crispy topping uses heart-healthy oats and nutrient-dense nuts. Use fresh berries in the summertime or frozen berries out of season.

Filling

6 cups mixed berries like blueberries, blackberries, raspberries, and strawberries (quartered)

¼ cup coconut palm sugar or

brown sugar

1 tablespoon lemon juice

3 tablespoons cornstarch

Topping

⅔ cup flour

⅓ cup coconut palm sugar or brown sugar

¼ teaspoon cinnamon

⅛ teaspoon salt

5 tablespoons cold unsalted butter, cut into small pieces

⅓ cup rolled oats

¼ cup chopped pecans or walnuts

Preheat oven to 375°F.

Toss the berries with the sugar, lemon juice, and cornstarch in a large bowl.

To make the topping, mix the flour, sugar, cinnamon, salt, and butter together in a stand mixer until the mixture is crumbly and sticks together in small clumps. Alternatively, you can use your hands to break the butter up and mix everything together in a bowl. Add the oats and nuts and mix until just combined.

Spray a 9-inch square baking dish with nonstick cooking spray and pour the berries and their juices into the dish. Spread the topping evenly over the fruit. Place the dish on a baking sheet (to catch any drippings) and bake in the oven until bubbly, 35 to 40 minutes. Cool 10 minutes before serving. Serve with vanilla ice cream or whipped cream.

NUTRITIONAL INFORMATION

One serving: Calories 259; Fat 9.8g (Sat 4.9g); Protein 3.7g; Carb 40g; Fiber 5.6g; Calcium 34mg; Iron 1.5mg; Sodium 3mg; Folate 53μg

---

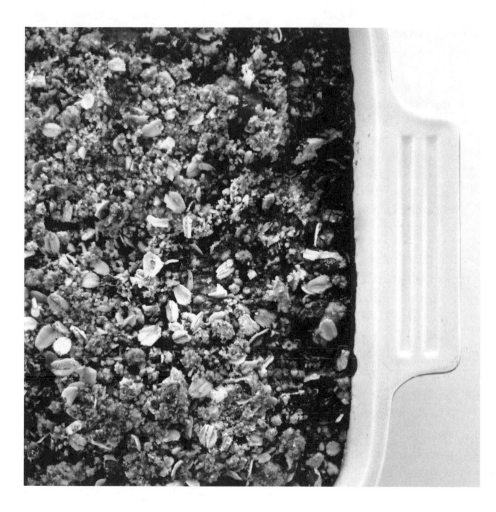

Cider Baked Apples

MAKES 4 SERVINGS

Celebrate fall's bounty with this mouthwatering apple dessert. This dish was created by my friend Ann at the Fountain Avenue Kitchen (www.fountainavenuekitchen.com). A crust-free version of the apple dumplings she grew up eating, these nutritious baked apples are brimming with whole grain oats, nutrient-packed nuts, and plenty of fiber. Ann suggests enjoying the leftovers for breakfast with some oatmeal.

4 apples (Granny Smith, Golden Delicious, Staymans, Fuji, etc.)
¼ cup rolled oats
¼ cup brown sugar
¼ cup unsweetened coconut
¼ cup chopped pecans or walnuts
1 teaspoon cinnamon
¼ teaspoon freshly grated nutmeg

4 teaspoons melted butter or coconut oil
1 cup pasteurized apple cider
Fresh cranberries or raisins (optional)
Toppings: Greek yogurt, whipped cream, or ice cream

Preheat the oven to 375°F. Slice a thin layer off the top of the apple (to hold more of the topping) and core, leaving about a half inch of the bottom intact. Set the apples in a pie plate or square baking dish. Then, mix the remaining ingredients except the butter and cider.

Stuff the holes with the oat mixture and mound slightly on top of the apples. Sprinkle a slightly rounded ¼ cup of the oat mixture around the bottom of the baking dish. This will help thicken the cider into a syrupy sauce. If using, scatter the fresh cranberries or raisins around the base of the baking dish.

Pour the cider around the apples (but not on top), and then top each apple with 1 teaspoon of butter or coconut oil. Cover the apples loosely with foil and bake for 20 minutes. Remove the foil and continue baking, about 10 to 20 minutes, or until you can poke a knife through the apple with no resistance.

Serve warm with a dollop of Greek yogurt, whipped cream, or ice cream, if desired.

NUTRITIONAL INFORMATION
One serving: Calories 302; Fat 10.7g (Sat 4.6g); Protein 3g; Carb 51.4g; Fiber 6.8g; Calcium 41mg; Iron 1.1mg; Sodium 20mg; Folate 12mg

Rock-a-Bye Baby Roasted Apricots

MAKES 4 SERVINGS

If you've never had fresh apricots, you must try this dish. Roasting apricots in the oven intensifies their sweet flavor and makes them meltingly tender and succulent. Apricots are rich in Vitamins A and C and are also a good source of fiber and potassium. These little gems are delicious on top of Greek yogurt or ice cream. They're also the perfect topping for a bowl of oatmeal in the morning along with some sliced almonds. They can even double as a nutritious treat for your baby. If you can't find fresh apricots, you can substitute nectarines, peaches, or plums and increase the cooking time.

1 pound fresh apricots (about 8 small apricots)
4 teaspoons brown sugar

⅛ teaspoon cinnamon
Vanilla Greek yogurt or ice cream

Preheat oven to 400°F. Cut the apricots in half and remove the seeds. Arrange the apricot halves in a cast-iron or other oven-safe skillet (you can also use a baking dish). Sprinkle the sugar and cinnamon evenly on top. Roast in the oven until apricots are softened, about 15 minutes. Serve apricots with vanilla Greek yogurt or ice cream. Spoon any pan juices on top.

NUTRITIONAL INFORMATION
One serving: Calories 65; Fat 0.3g (Sat 0g); Protein 1.6g; Carb 15.6g; Fiber 2.3g; Calcium 17mg; Iron 0.5mg; Sodium 1mg; Folate 10μg

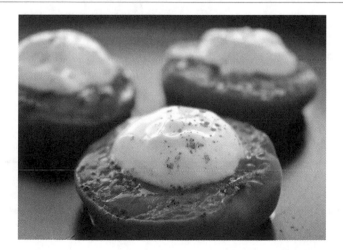

Fresh Strawberry Cake

MAKES 8 SERVINGS

This cake is bursting with beautiful, fresh strawberries that give it a lovely presentation. It's easy to make, and you can serve it to guests, right from the pie plate—it doesn't get much better than that! Strawberries supply plenty of antioxidants, Vitamin C, and fiber. The addition of white whole wheat flour adds a dose of whole grains and Greek yogurt gives a protein boost. Serve the cake alone or with a dollop of freshly whipped cream.

1 cup all-purpose flour
½ cup white whole wheat flour
1½ teaspoons baking powder
½ teaspoon salt
6 tablespoons unsalted butter or coconut oil
¾ cup sugar plus 2 teaspoons, divided
1 large egg

⅓ cup whole or 2% milk
¼ cup vanilla nonfat Greek yogurt
1 teaspoon vanilla
1 teaspoon lemon zest
12 ounces organic strawberries, stemmed and halved
Optional topping: freshly whipped cream

Preheat oven to 350°F. Spray a 9-inch pie plate with cooking spray. Whisk the flours, baking powder, and salt together into a medium bowl. Beat the butter and ¾ cup sugar together in the bowl of a stand mixer fitted with a paddle attachment. Mix on medium-high speed until pale yellow and fluffy, about 2 minutes. Reduce speed to medium and add the egg, milk, yogurt, vanilla, and lemon zest. Reduce speed to low and slowly add in the flour mixture. Mix until just incorporated (do not over-mix).

Transfer the batter to the prepared pie plate and smooth out the top with a spatula. Arrange the strawberries on top of the batter, cut side down, packing them in as closely as possible. Sprinkle the remaining 2 teaspoons sugar over the top. Bake until cake is golden and a toothpick inserted into the center comes out clean. Cool on a wire rack. Cut into wedges and serve alone or with freshly whipped cream.

NUTRITIONAL INFORMATION
One serving: Calories 266; Fat 9.2g (Sat 5.9g); Protein 4.1g; Carb 41.4g; Fiber 2.1g; Calcium 79mg; Iron 1.4mg; Sodium 251mg; Folate 45mg

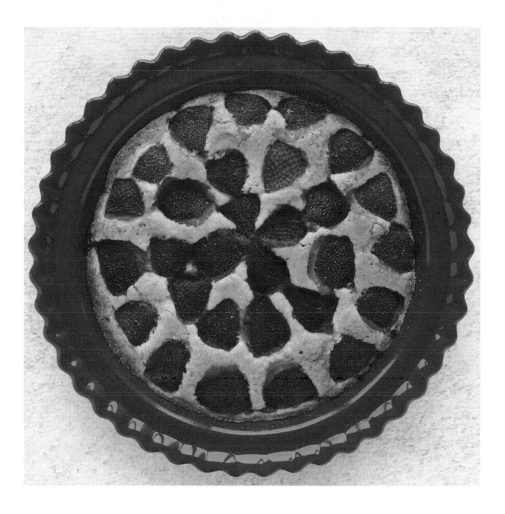

Craveable Chocolate Ganache Cupcakes

MAKES 12 CUPCAKES

Who says you can't have your cake and eat it, too? Let's face it; sometimes we all need a chocolate fix. Rather than deny yourself, practice portion control by diving into one of these rich, moist cupcakes. At less than 250 calories apiece, these chocolaty treats will satisfy your cravings and you can feel good about it. Plus, chocolate is packed with flavonoids, powerful antioxidants. Not all chocolates are equal though so reach for dark chocolate over milk chocolate as it has the highest amount of these important nutrients.

Ganache
5 ounces dark chocolate chips (about ¾ cup)

⅓ cup heavy cream

Cupcakes
¾ cup plus 2 tablespoons enriched all-purpose flour
1 cup sugar
6 tablespoons cocoa powder
¾ teaspoons baking powder
¾ teaspoons baking soda
¼ teaspoon salt
1 large egg

½ cup whole milk
¼ cup neutral-flavored oil like safflower or vegetable oil
1 teaspoon vanilla
½ cup boiling water
Optional toppings: shredded coconut, chocolate chips, or sliced almonds

Preheat oven to 350°F. To make the ganache, place the chocolate chips in a large bowl. Heat the cream in a small saucepan until just boiling. Immediately pour the cream over the chocolate chips. Cover the bowl and let it sit for a few minutes to melt the chocolate. Slowly stir the mixture using a rubber spatula until the chocolate is completely melted and a smooth sauce forms, about 2 minutes. Let the ganache cool while you make the cupcakes. As it cools, it will thicken.

To make the cupcakes, whisk the flour, sugar, cocoa powder, baking powder, baking soda, and salt together in a large bowl. Add the egg, milk, oil, and vanilla and mix the ingredients together with a hand mixer until smooth. Pour in the water and continue to mix until incorporated. The batter will be thin.

Line a 12-cup muffin pan with paper liners. Pour the batter into the cups, filling them about ¾ full. Bake in the oven for 22 to 24 minutes, until a toothpick inserted into the center of the cupcakes comes out clean. Cool completely.

Frost the cupcakes with the cooled ganache. Serve plain or garnish with desired toppings like shredded coconut, chocolate chips, or sliced almonds.

NUTRITIONAL INFORMATION
One cupcake: Calories 247; Fat 11.8g (Sat 8.4g); Protein 3.2g; Carb 32.2g; Fiber 2.1g; Calcium 47mg; Iron 1.7mg; Sodium 172mg; Folate 30mg

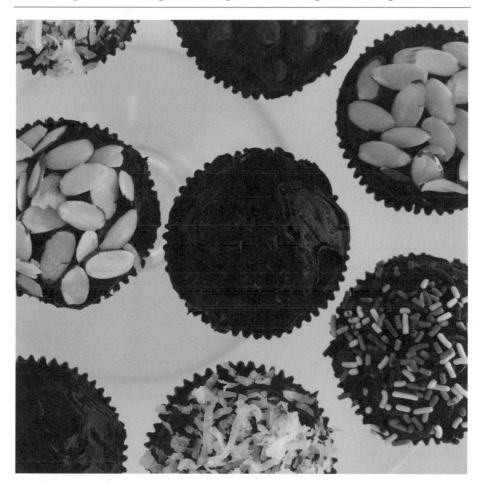

Flourless Peanut Butter Cookies

MAKES 1 DOZEN COOKIES

Here's an easy, family-friendly cookie recipe shared by my friend Lauren from Lauren Kelly Nutrition (www.laurenkellynutrition.com). These delicious, gluten-free peanut butter cookies provide plenty of protein and fiber as well as a boost of omega-3 fatty acids from flaxseed. Satisfying and delicious, they're the ideal snack when you're craving something sweet. Although they're perfect as is, if you're a chocolate fan, Lauren suggests adding some chocolate chips to make them even more perfect.

½ cup natural peanut butter
¼ cup honey
3 tablespoons coconut oil, softened
2 cage-free eggs, beaten
1 teaspoon pure vanilla extract

¼ cup rolled oats
½ teaspoon baking soda
1 teaspoon cinnamon
¼ teaspoon sea salt
3 tablespoons ground flaxseed

Preheat oven to 350°F. Mix the peanut butter, honey, and coconut oil until combined. Add the eggs and vanilla and mix until incorporated. Add the oats, baking soda, cinnamon, salt, and flaxseed and mix until well combined. Place by spoonfuls onto a baking sheet lined with a silicone baking mat or parchment paper. Bake in oven for 12 to 15 minutes until edges are golden brown.

NUTRITIONAL INFORMATION
One cookie: Calories 147; Fat 9.9g (Sat 4.4g); Protein 4.5g; Carb 10.9g; Fiber 1.6g; Calcium 17mg; Iron 0.6mg; Sodium 113mg; Folate 14mg

Honey Lemon Cookies

MAKES 32 COOKIES

These delightful little lemon cookies were shared by my friend Christie from Food Done Light (www.fooddonelight.com). To make them healthier, she incorporates whole wheat flour, which supplies plenty of vitamins, minerals, and fiber. Greek yogurt adds moisture and a boost of protein while the honey provides natural sweetness. Arrange these adorable confections on a platter and serve them as a light dessert.

½ cup sugar
4 tablespoons unsalted butter, softened
3 tablespoons light butter, softened
2 teaspoons lemon zest
⅓ cup honey
½ teaspoon lemon extract
1 large egg, at room temperature
1¼ cups unbleached, all-purpose flour
½ cup whole wheat pastry flour
1 teaspoon baking powder
½ teaspoon kosher salt
¼ cup plain nonfat Greek yogurt
1 cup powdered sugar
2 tablespoons lemon juice
Optional: sprinkles or lemon zest for decoration

Preheat oven to 350°F. In the bowl of a stand mixer, combine sugar, butter, and lemon zest. Beat until light and fluffy, about 5 minutes. Add honey, lemon extract, and egg and beat until well combined.

In a medium bowl, whisk together all-purpose flour, whole wheat flour, baking powder, and salt. Add one-third of the flour mixture to the wet ingredients and beat until incorporated. Stir in half of the yogurt. Repeat with the remaining flour and yogurt, ending with the last third of the flour.

Line two baking sheets with parchment paper or silicone baking mat. Drop level tablespoons of batter onto the cookie sheet, leaving a 2-inch border between the cookies. Bake about 12 minutes or until cookies are lightly brown.

While cookies are baking, make the glaze by whisking the powdered sugar and lemon juice together. As soon as the cookies come out of the oven, use a pastry brush to paint on the glaze. Sprinkle immediately with lemon zest or sprinkles, if using. Transfer cookies to a wire rack and cool completely.

NUTRITIONAL INFORMATION
One cookie: Calories 82; Fat 2.2g (Sat 1.4g); Protein 1.1g; Carb 14.5g; Fiber 0.4g; Calcium 15mg; Iron 0.4mg; Sodium 56mg; Folate 16mg

Buttermilk Blueberry Scookies

MAKES 12–14 SCOOKIES

My friend Ally, the creative mind behind Ally's Kitchen (www.allyskitchen.com), developed this wonderful recipe that's a cross between a scone and a cookie. This adventurous lady is a mother, and grandmother and she describes her style of cooking (and living) as "Bohemian Bold". Equally delicious for dessert or breakfast, these scookies can be served plain or topped with a fruit sauce like Blueberry Maple Compote (page 87). This dish provides antioxidants and folate.

2 cups all-purpose flour
½ cup sugar (plus 1 tablespoon), divided
2 teaspoons baking powder
1 teaspoon baking soda

½ cup cold salted butter, cut in cubes
1 egg, beaten
½ cup reduced-fat buttermilk
1 cup fresh blueberries

Preheat oven to 375°F. Sift the flour, ½ cup sugar, baking powder, and baking soda into a large mixing bowl. Add the butter cubes, and with your hands or a pastry cutter, blend into the flour mixture.

In a small bowl, combine the egg and buttermilk. Pour into the dry mixture and mix well. The batter will be thick. Dollop the batter onto a baking sheet lined with parchment paper. You should have 12–14 scookies. Take a teaspoon, coat the back with cooking spray, and use this to make an indentation in the center of each one. Place some blueberries in each one and gently press them down into the centers. Sprinkle with the remaining tablespoon sugar. Bake in the oven for 10 to 12 minutes or until the scookies are golden brown.

NUTRITIONAL INFORMATION
One scookie: Calories 183; Fat 7.3g (Sat 4.8g); Protein 3; Carb 25.7g; Fiber 0.8g; Calcium 62mg; Iron 1.1mg; Sodium 248mg; Folate 59mg

Super-Fast Peach Frozen Yogurt

MAKES 4 SERVINGS

Did you know you can make your own frozen yogurt at home? This family-friendly treat is nutritious, delicious, and takes only five minutes to make. Peaches supply a rich dose of Vitamin C and Greek yogurt adds a boost of protein and calcium.

16 ounces frozen sliced peaches (do not defrost)
½ cup vanilla low-fat or nonfat Greek yogurt

3–4 tablespoons honey or sweetener of your choice (adjust to taste)
1 tablespoon fresh lemon juice

Place all of the ingredients into the bowl of a large food processor. Blend, scraping down the sides occasionally, until it forms a creamy, smooth mixture. This should take about 4 to 5 minutes. At this point the frozen yogurt can be served and will have the texture of soft serve. For a firmer texture, transfer the mixture to a freezer container and freeze for an hour or two before serving.

NUTRITIONAL INFORMATION
One serving: Calories 122; Fat 0.6g (Sat 0.3g); Protein 2.8g; Carb 29g; Fiber 1.7g; Calcium 68mg; Iron 0.4mg; Sodium 23mg; Folate 9mg

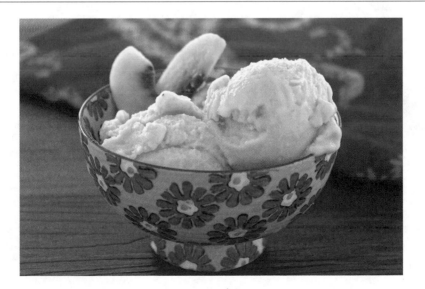

One-Ingredient Banana Ice Cream

MAKES 4 SERVINGS

The next time you get a serious ice cream craving, try this dish—it's quick, easy and nutritious and you don't even need an ice cream maker! It's hard to believe, but when you blend chopped up frozen bananas in a food processor, the result is a deliciously rich and creamy treat that tastes like soft serve ice cream. This dairy-free ice cream is rich in fiber as well as Vitamin B_6, Vitamin C, potassium, and manganese.

4 ripe bananas, peeled

Cut the bananas into 1-inch pieces. Put them on a plate in a single layer and freeze until solid, at least 1 to 2 hours or overnight. Place the frozen banana pieces in a food processor. Puree until creamy, about 2 to 3 minutes, scraping down the sides as needed. The ice cream can be served at this point and will have a texture similar to soft serve ice cream. For a firmer texture, transfer the ice cream to an airtight container and place it in the freezer for at least an hour. Let the ice cream soften for about 10 minutes before serving.

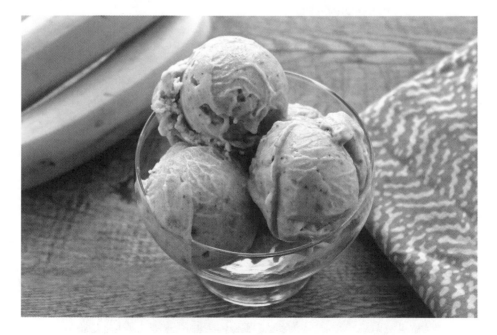

Banana Peanut Butter Ice Cream

Add 2 tablespoons peanut butter to the ice cream and blend.

Chunky Monkey Ice Cream

Stir 2 tablespoons dark chocolate chips and 2 tablespoons chopped walnuts into the ice cream.

Banana Nutella Ice Cream

Add ¼ cup Nutella to the ice cream and blend.

Banana Berry Ice Cream

Freeze 2 cups chopped strawberries with the bananas. Puree together in a food processor with ⅓ cup low-fat milk.

NUTRITIONAL INFORMATION
One serving: Calories 105; Fat 0.3g (Sat 0.1g); Protein 1.3g; Carb 27g; Fiber 3.1g; Calcium 5mg; Iron 0.3mg; Sodium 1mg; Folate 23mg

Lemon Raspberry Buttermilk Popsicles

MAKES 8 POPSICLES

Popsicles are a great way to stay hydrated and get a healthy dose of nutrients on days when you're not feeling up to eating. Buttermilk provides protein and calcium, while raspberries add antioxidants, Vitamin C, and fiber. As an added bonus, the lemon juice may help alleviate nausea.

1½ cups reduced-fat buttermilk
4 tablespoons fresh lemon juice
4 tablespoons honey or sweetener of your choice
1 cup raspberries

Whisk the buttermilk, lemon juice, and honey together in a bowl. Pour the mixture into eight 3-ounce popsicle molds. Place the raspberries in a bowl and crush them with a fork until pureed. Spoon equal amounts of the raspberry puree into the popsicle molds. Using a chopstick, carefully push the raspberry puree down into the buttermilk mixture, trying not to mix it in too much (if you mix it too much, the popsicles will turn pink). Place the popsicle sticks into the popsicles, cover and freeze for 2 to 3 hours, until solid. Alternatively, if you don't have popsicle molds, you can use small paper cups.

To unmold, dip the popsicle molds in warm water and then pull the popsicles out. Enjoy!

NUTRITIONAL INFORMATION
One serving: Calories 67; Fat 0.9g (Sat 0.6g); Protein 2.1g; Carb 13.5g; Fiber 1g; Calcium 70mg; Iron 0.2mg; Sodium 40mg; Folate 7mg

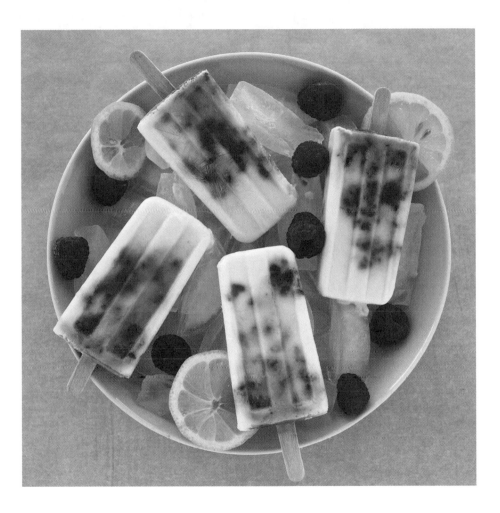

Cherry Lime Granita

MAKES 4 SERVINGS

This dish just sings summer! An incredibly refreshing dessert, a granita is basically like a grown-up slushy and is a great way to beat the heat. It requires no special equipment and is made by freezing a flavored liquid or puree in a shallow container and scraping it with a fork occasionally to give it a flaky consistency. Cherries are packed with antioxidants and also supply considerable fiber and Vitamin C.

1 bag (12 ounces) frozen, pitted cherries (or fresh)
1 cup cold water
4 teaspoons sugar, honey, or sweetener of your choice (adjust to taste)

1 tablespoon lime juice
Optional garnishes: whipped cream, lime zest

Blend all ingredients together in a blender. Adjust sweetness to taste. Pour the mixture into a shallow glass baking dish and place in the freezer.

Remove the dish after 30 minutes. Using a fork, scrape the mixture, breaking up any icy clumps. Return the dish to the freezer. Repeat the process every thirty minutes or so, scraping the mixture with a fork to break up the ice crystals and create a light and fluffy texture. It should take about 2 hours total.

Scoop the granita into dessert bowls. Serve plain or garnish with whipped cream and/or lime zest. Serve immediately.

NUTRITIONAL INFORMATION

One serving: Calories 79; Fat 0.1g (Sat 0g); Protein 1.1g; Carb 20.4g; Fiber 2.1g; Calcium 15mg; Iron 0.4mg; Sodium 1mg; Folate 4mg

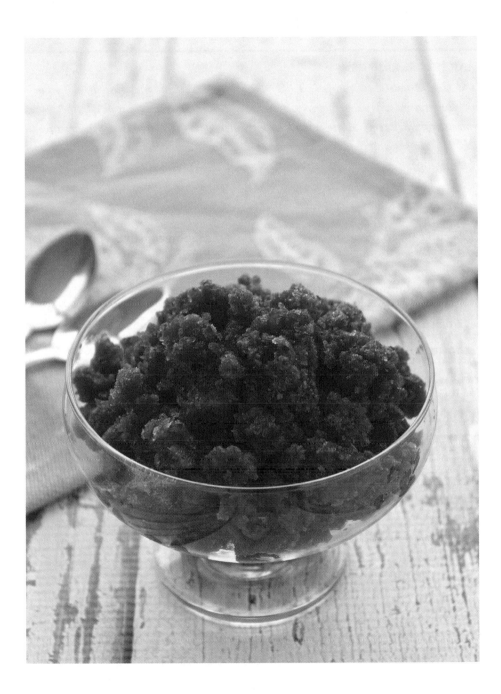

Pumpkin Custard

MAKES 4 SERVINGS

This elegant dessert, which is just like pumpkin pie without the crust, is sure to be a hit! This recipe was shared by my friend Amee over at Amee's Savory Dish (www. ameessavorydish.com). Amee is a mom, a trainer and a self-described Southern foodie who loves to eat and create healthy recipe makeovers. You'll get plenty of nutrients with this dish including protein, Vitamin A, Vitamin C, Vitamin K, and calcium. She notes that the key to this recipe is to sift the sugar mixture before adding it to the other ingredients to ensure a silky smooth texture.

¾ cup canned pumpkin puree
2 large eggs
1½ cups whole milk
1 teaspoon vanilla extract
½ cup coconut palm sugar
2 teaspoons cornstarch

½ teaspoon cinnamon plus extra for garnish
¼ teaspoon pumpkin pie spice
¼ teaspoon sea salt
Optional toppings: whipped cream, chopped pecans

Preheat oven to 350°F. In a large bowl, whisk together the pumpkin, eggs, milk, and vanilla. In another bowl, stir together the coconut sugar, cornstarch, spices, and sea salt. Sift sugar mixture into the pumpkin mixture. Stir the batter with a whisk until combined well and pour into four ¾-cup custard cups. Place cups in a 9 x 11-inch baking pan and add enough warm water to come halfway up the sides of the cups.

Bake in the oven for 50 minutes, or until it sets and is lightly browned. Transfer cups to a wire rack to cool. Top with a little whipped cream and sprinkle with cinnamon.

NUTRITIONAL INFORMATION
One serving: Calories 220; Fat 4.9g (Sat 2.6g); Protein 6.6g; Carb 37.1g; Fiber 1.5g; Calcium 155mg; Iron 1.4mg; Sodium 229mg; Folate 22mg

APPENDIX A:

KNOW YOUR BMI

BMI

BMI, which stands for body mass index, is a measure of body fat based on your weight and height. Once you know your BMI, you can see which weight category you fall into.

BMI	CLASSIFICATION
<18.5	Underweight
18.5–24.9	Normal weight
25.0–29.9	Overweight
>30	Obese

You can calculate your BMI using the equation below or look up your BMI on the chart below.

Calculate your BMI

MEASUREMENT UNITS	BMI FORMULA
Kilograms and meters (or centimeters)	weight (kg) / [height (m)]^2
Pounds and inches	weight (lb) / [height (in)]^2 x 703

Look up your BMI

Body Mass Index (BMI) Chart

WEIGHT	lbs	100	105	110	115	120	125	130	135	140	145	150	155	160	165	170	175	180	185	190	195	200	205	210	215
	kgs	45.4	47.6	49.9	52.2	54.4	56.7	59.0	61.2	63.5	65.8	68.0	70.3	72.6	74.8	77.1	79.4	81.6	83.9	86.2	88.5	90.7	93.0	95.3	97.5
HEIGHT ft/in	cm																								
5'0"	152.4	19	20	21	22	23	24	25	26	27	28	29	30	31	32	33	34	35	36	37	38	39	40	41	42
5'1"	154.9	18	19	20	21	22	23	24	25	26	27	28	29	30	31	32	33	34	35	36	36	37	38	39	40
5'2"	157.5	18	19	20	21	22	22	23	24	25	26	27	28	29	30	31	32	33	33	34	35	36	37	38	39
5'3"	160.0	17	18	19	20	21	22	23	24	24	25	26	27	28	29	30	31	32	32	33	34	35	36	37	38
5'4"	162.6	17	18	18	19	20	21	22	23	24	24	25	26	27	28	29	30	31	31	32	33	34	35	36	37
5'5"	165.1	16	17	18	19	20	20	21	22	23	24	25	25	26	27	28	29	30	30	31	32	33	34	35	35
5'6"	167.6	16	17	17	18	19	20	21	21	22	23	24	25	25	26	27	28	29	29	30	31	32	33	34	34
5'7"	170.2	15	16	17	18	18	19	20	21	22	22	23	24	25	25	26	27	28	29	29	30	31	32	33	33
5'8"	172.7	15	16	16	17	18	19	19	20	21	22	22	23	24	25	25	26	27	28	28	29	30	31	32	32
5'9"	175.3	14	15	16	17	17	18	19	20	20	21	22	22	23	24	25	25	26	27	28	28	29	30	31	31
5'10"	177.8	14	15	16	16	17	18	18	19	20	20	21	22	23	23	24	25	25	26	27	28	28	29	30	30
5'11"	180.3	14	14	15	16	16	17	18	18	19	20	21	21	22	23	23	24	25	25	26	27	28	28	29	30
6'0"	182.9	13	14	14	15	16	17	17	18	19	19	20	21	21	22	23	23	24	25	25	26	27	27	28	29
6'1"	185.4	13	13	14	15	15	16	17	17	18	19	19	20	21	21	22	23	23	24	25	25	26	27	27	28
6'2"	188.0	12	13	14	14	15	16	16	17	18	18	19	19	20	21	21	22	23	23	24	25	25	26	27	27
6'3"	190.5	12	13	13	14	15	15	16	16	17	18	18	19	20	20	21	21	22	23	23	24	25	25	26	26
6'4"	193.0	12	12	13	14	14	15	15	16	17	17	18	18	19	20	20	21	22	22	23	23	24	25	25	26

Underweight   Ideal   Overweight   Obese   Extremely obese

APPENDIX B:

DIETARY REFERENCE INTAKES FOR PREGNANCY AND BREASTFEEDING

Dietary reference intakes (DRIs) are the recommended amounts an individual should consume daily of certain nutrients, vitamins, and minerals.

NUTRIENT	PREGNANT AGE 18 YEARS AND YOUNGER	PREGNANT AGE 19 TO 50 YEARS	BREASTFEEDING AGE 18 YEARS AND YOUNGER	BREASTFEEDING AGE 19 TO 50 YEARS
Protein (g)	71	71	71	71
Carbohydrates(g)	175	175	210	210
Fiber (g)	28	28	29	29
Vitamin A (mg)	750	770	1,200	1,300
Vitamin D (mg/IU)	5/200	5/200	5/200	5/200
Vitamin E (mg)	15	15	19	19
Vitamin K (mg)	75	90	75	90
Vitamin C (mg)	80	85	115	120
Thiamin (mg)	1.4	1.4	1.4	1.4
Riboflavin (mg)	1.4	1.4	1.6	1.6
Niacin (mg)	18	18	17	17
Vitamin B_6 (mg)	1.9	1.9	2.0	2.0
Folate (mg)	600	600	500	500
Vitamin B_{12} (mg)	2.6	2.6	2.8	2.8
Iron (mg)	27	27	10	9
Calcium (mg)	1,300	1,000	1,300	1,000
Phosphorus (mg)	1,250	700	1,250	700
Magnesium (mg)	400	360	360	320
Zinc (mg)	12	11	13	12
Iodine (mg)	220	220	290	290
Biotin (mg)	30	30	35	35
Choline (mg)	450	450	550	550
Selenium (mg)	60	60	70	70
Sodium (mg)	1,500	1,500	1,500	1,500
Potassium (mg)	4,700	4,700	5,100	5,100

PREGNANCY RESOURCES

Academy of Nutrition and Dietetics
www.eatright.org

American Congress of Obstetricians and Gynecologists
www.acog.org

American Diabetes Association
www.diabetes.org

Environmental Working Group
www.ewg.org/foodnews/index.php

Food Safety
www.usda.gov/wps/portal/usda/usdahome?navid=food-safety

National Women's Health Information Center
www.womenshealth.gov

Special Supplemental Nutrition Program for Women,
Infants, and Children (WIC)
Food and Nutrition Service
www.fns.usda.gov/wic

Super Tracker
www.supertracker.usda.gov

USDA Dietary Guidelines for Americans
www.cnpp.usda.gov/DGAs2010-PolicyDocument.htm

USDA MyPlate: Health and Nutrition Information
for Pregnant and Breastfeeding Women
www.choosemyplate.gov/pregnancy-breastfeeding.html

REFERENCES

Introduction

1. Adams, Kelly M. MPH, RD; Kohlmeier, Martin MD; Zeisel, Steven H. MD, PhD. (2010). Nutrition Education in U.S. Medical Schools: Latest Update of a National Survey. *Academic Medicine*, 85(9), 1537–1542.

Chapter 1

1. Institute of Medicine. Weight gain during pregnancy: reexamining the guidelines. Washington, DC: National Academies Press; 2009.

2. Siega-Riz, AM, Viswanathan, M, Moos, MK, Deierlein, A, Mumford, S, Knaack, J, et al. A systematic review of outcomes of maternal weight gain according to the Institute of Medicine recommendations: Birthweight, fetal growth, and postpartum weight retention. *Am J Obstet Gynecol* 2009; 201:339.e1–14.

3. Oken, E, Taveras, EM, Kleinman, KP, Rich-Edwards, JW, and Gillman, MW. Gestational weight gain and child adiposity at age 3 years. *Am J Obstet* Gynecol. 2007; 196:322.e1–322.e8.

4. Olson CM, Strawderman MS, and Dennison BA, Maternal weight gain during pregnancy and child weight at age 3 years. *Matern Child Health J.* 2009; 13:839–846. Epub 2008 Sep 26.

5. Jones, C and Hudson, R. *Eating for Pregnancy: The essential nutrition guide and cookbook for today's mothers-to-be,* 2nd edition. Cambridge: Da Capo Press, 2009.

6. Staying healthy and safe. Office on Women's Health, US Dept of Health and Human Services. http://www.womenshealth.gov

7. Lammi-Keefe, C, Couch, S, Philipson, E, editors. *Handbook of Nutrition and Pregnancy.* Totowa, NJ: Humana Press, 2008.

8. Grosvenor, M and Smolin, L. *Visualizing Nutrition: Everyday Choices,* 2nd Edition. Hoboken, NJ: John Wiley & Sons, 2012.

9. Whole Grains Council. Wholegrainscouncil.org

10. Coletta, J, Bell, S, and Roman, A. Omega-3 Fatty Acids and Pregnancy. *Rev Obstet Gynecol* 2010 Fall; 3(4): 163–171.

11. Helland, IB, Smith, L, Saarem, K, et al. Maternal supplementation with very-long-chain n-3 fatty acids during pregnancy and lactation augments children's IQ at 4 years of age. *Pediatrics* 2003111:e39–e44.

12. Makrides, M, Gibson, RA, McPhee, AJ, et al. Effect of DHA supplementation during pregnancy on maternal depression and neurodevelopment of young children: a randomized controlled trial. *JAMA* 2010; 304:1675–1683.

13. Furuhjelm, C, Warstedt, K, Larsson, J, et al. Fish oil supplementation in pregnancy and lactation may decrease the risk of infant allergy. *Acta Paediatr* 2009;98:1461–1467.

14. Scholl, TO and Johnson WG. Folic acid: influence on the outcome of pregnancy. *Am J Clin Nutr* 2000; 71(5 Suppl); 1295S–1303S.

15. Berry, RJ, Bailey, L, Mulinaire, J, and Bower, C. Fortification of flour with folic acid. *Food Nutr Bull* 2010; 31 (1 Suppl.) S22-S35, 2010.

16. De Wals, P, Tiarou, F, Van Allen, MI, et al. Reduction in neural-tube defects after folic acid fortification in Canada. *N Engl J Med* 2007; 357:135–142.

17. World Health Organization. Iron Deficiency Anaemia: Assessment, Prevention, and Control, 2001. Who.int/nutrition/publications/en/ida_assessment_prevention_control.pdf

18. Quintaes KD, Farfan JA, Tomazini FM, and Morgano MA. Mineral migration from stainless steel, cast-iron, and soapstone (steatite) Brazilian pans to food preparations. *Arch Latinoam Nutr* 2006 Sep;56(3):275–81.

19. World Health Organization (WHO). WHO recommendations for prevention and treatment of pre-eclampsia and eclampsia. Geneva (Switzerland): World Health Organization (WHO); 2011.

Chapter 2

1. Daily food plan for moms. U.S. Department of Agriculture. Choosemyplate.gov/supertracker-tools/daily-food-plans/moms.html

2. The Vegetarian Resource Group. Vrg.org/journal/.

3. DeSisto, CL, Kim, SY, and Sharma, AJ. Prevalence Estimates of Gestational Diabetes Mellitus in the United States, Pregnancy Risk Assessment Monitoring System (PRAMS), 2007–2010. *Prev Chronic Dis* 2014;11:130415.

Chapter 3

1. The American College of Obstetricians and Gynecologists. *Your Pregnancy and Childbirth: Month to Month*, 5th Edition. Washington, DC: ACOG, 2010.

2. Steele, NM, French, J, Gatherer-Boyles, J, et al. Effect of acupressure by Sea-Bands on nausea and vomiting of pregnancy. *Obstet Gynecol Neonatal Nurs*. 2001 Jan-Feb;30(1):61–70.

3. Barclay, Laurie. ACOG Guidelines for Treating Nausea and Vomiting in Pregnant Women Reviewed. Medscape.com, 2010.

4. Niebyl, J. Nausea and Vomiting in Pregnancy. *N Engl J Med* 2010; 363:1544–50.

5. Jednak, MA, Shadigian, EM, Kim, MS, et al. Protein meals reduce nausea and gastric slow wave dysrhythmic activity in first trimester pregnancy. *Am J Physiol* 1999;277:G855.

6. Smith, JA, Refuerzo Jerrie, and S, Ramin, Susan M. Treatment and outcome of nausea and vomiting of pregnancy. Uptodate.com, 2014.

Chapter 4

1. Cdc.gov

2. Foodsafety.adcouncil.org

3. Fsis.usda.gov

4. Fda.gov

5. Rauch, S, Braun, J, Boyd, D, et al. Associations of Prenatal Exposure to Organophosphate Pesticide Metabolites with Gestational Age and Birth Weight. *Environ Health Perspect* Jul 2012; 120(7): 1055–1060.

6. Policy Statement by the American Academy of Pediatrics: Pesticide Exposure in Children. *Pediatrics* 2012; 130(6):1757–1763.

7. Bouchard, A, Chevrier, J, Harley, K, et al. Prenatal Exposure to Organophosphate Pesticides and IQ in 7-Year-Old Children. *Environ Health Perspect*. 2011 August; 119(8): 1189–1195.

8. Engel, S, Wetmur, J, Chen, J et al. Prenatal Exposure to Organophosphates, Paraoxonase 1, and Cognitive Development in Childhood. *Environ Health Perspect*. 2011 August; 119(8): 1182–1188.

9. Rauh, V, Arunajadai, S, Horton, M, et al. Seven-Year Neurodevelopmental Scores and Prenatal Exposure to Chlorpyrifos, a Common Agricultural Pesticide. *Environ Health Perspect*. 2011 August; 119(8): 1196–1201.

10. The American College of Obstetricians & Gynecologists Committee on Opinion. Moderate Caffeine Consumption During Pregnancy. *Obstetrics & Gynecology*, August 2010; 116: pp 467–468.

11. Acog.org

12. Stratton, K, Howe, C, and Battaglia F, editors. Committee to Study Fetal Alcohol Syndrome, Institute of Medicine. Fetal Alcohol Syndrome: Diagnosis, Epidemiology, Prevention, and Treatment. Washington, DC: Institute of Medicine, National Academy Press, 1996.

13. Augustin, J, Augustin, E, Cutrufelli RL, et al. Alcohol Retention in Food Preparation. *J Am Diet Assoc*1992;92:486-488.

Chapter 5

1. Bayol, S; Farrington, S; Stickland, N. A. Maternal "junk food" diet in pregnancy and lactation promotes an exacerbated taste for "junk food" and a greater propensity for obesity in rat offspring. *Br J Nutr* 2007; 98(4),843–851.

2. Kerver, JM, et al. Meal and snack patterns are associated with dietary intake of energy and nutrients in U.S. adults. *J Am Diet Assoc* 2006;106:46.

3. Gibson, SA, et al. What's for breakfast? Nutritional implications of breakfast habits: Insights from the NDNS dietary records. *Nutr Bull* 2011;36:78.

4. Institute of Medicine of the National Academies. Dietary Reference Intakes: Water, Potassium, Sodium, Chloride, and Sulfate. Iom.edu/Reports/2004/Dietary-Reference-Intakes-Water-Potassium-Sodium-Chloride-and-Sulfate.aspx

5. Office of Disease Prevention and Health Promotion. 2008 Physical Activity Guidelines for Americans. Health.gov/paguidelines.

INDEX

A

Acorn Squash, Maple-Glazed, 227
acupressure wrist bands, 31
adobo
    Pumpkin Turkey Chili, 187–188
Agua Fresca, Watermelon, 139–140
ALA (alpha-linolenic acid), 15–16
Alaskan seafood, purity of, 43
alcohol, foods to avoid or limit, 48
Alcoholic Beverage Labeling Act, 48
Ally's Kitchen, 254
almond butter
    Banana Nut Health Shake, 137
Almond Chia Pudding with
    Raspberries, 92
Almond Joy No-Cook Overnight
    Oats, 95
almond milk
    Almond Chia Pudding with
        Raspberries, 92
    Almond Joy No-Cook Overnight
        Oats, 95
    Banana Nut Health Shake, 137
    Blueberry Vanilla No-Cook
        Overnight Oats, 94
    Nutty Nana No-Cook Overnight
        Oats, 95
    Peachy-Keen Baked Oatmeal, 84
    Strawberry Almond Breakfast
        Quinoa, 90
almonds
    Almond Joy No-Cook Overnight
        Oats, 95
    No-Bake Chocolate Cherry
        Granola Bars, 110–111
    Quinoa Salad with Spinach,
        Strawberries, and Goat Cheese,
        159–160
    Strawberry Almond Breakfast
        Quinoa, 90
    White Gazpacho, 151
alpha-linolenic acid (ALA), 15–16
Amee's Savory Dish, 262
anchovy paste
    Pantry Pasta Puttanesca, 212
anemia, iron-deficiency, 18, 33
appetizers, snacks, and sandwiches
    Avocado Toast, 112
    Black Bean and Quinoa Veggie
        Burgers, 126–128
    Brain-Boosting Salmon Burgers,
        125–126
    Cauliflower Cheesy Bread, 104
    Chili Lime Avocado Toast, 112
    Chipotle Burgers with Avocado
        Crema, 128–129
    Crispy Kale Chips, 119
    Crispy Spiced Chickpeas, 116
    Deviled Egg Spread, 118

Feta and Radish Avocado Toast,
    113
Greek Chicken Meatballs, 107
Green Grilled Cheese Sandwich,
    131
Homemade Vegan Mayonnaise,
    123–124
No-Bake Chocolate Cherry
    Granola Bars, 110–111
Pan con Tomate (Tomato Bread),
    106
Quick Pickled Shallots, 123
Refrigerator Dill Pickles, 117
Roasted Sweet Potato and Black
    Bean Tacos, 210–211
Roasted Vegetable Hummus
    Wraps, 124
Sesame Noodles with Broccoli, 108
Simply Delicious Hummus, 114
Snack Attack Spiced Nuts, 122
Spanish Garlic Shrimp (Gambas al
    Ajillo), 102
Tropical Popcorn Trail Mix, 120
Turkey Parmesan Burgers, 130
Turkey Sausage Egg White
    Flatbread, 79–80
Wok-Charred Edamame with
    Sweet Soy Glaze, 100
Apple Cinnamon Dutch Baby, 74
apples
    Apple Cinnamon Dutch Baby, 74
    Autumn Celery Root Puree, 230
    Cider Baked Apples, 246
    Tuscan Kale and Apple Salad,
        154–155
appliance thermometers, 41
Apricots, Rock-a-Bye Baby Roasted,
    247
artichoke hearts
    Mediterranean Shrimp Pasta, 176
arugula
    Crispy Chicken with Tomato
        Arugula Salad, 182–183
    Roasted Butternut Squash Salad
        with Maple Dijon Vinaigrette,
        160–161
asparagus
    Roasted Asparagus and Grape
        Tomatoes with Balsamic and
        Pecorino, 231
Autumn Celery Root Puree, 230
avocados
    Avocado Toast, 112
    Chili Lime Avocado Toast, 112
    Chipotle Burgers with Avocado
        Crema, 128–129
    Feta and Radish Avocado Toast,
        113

Green Grilled Cheese Sandwich,
    131
Roasted Sweet Potato and Black
    Bean Tacos, 180
Tropical Shrimp Salad, 162–163
Avocado Toast, 112

B

Baby Bellini, 140–141
Baby Bump Banana Flax Bread, 73
Baby on Board Blueberry Peach
    Cobbler, 242–243
background of book, v–vii, 67
bacon
    Cheesy Quinoa and Bacon
        Casserole, 203
bacteria in food. see food safety
baking ingredients, essential, 60
Balsamic, Maple, and Thyme Roasted
    Chicken, 194–195
balsamic vinegar
    Balsamic Dressing, 159–160
    Balsamic, Maple, and Thyme
        Roasted Chicken, 194–195
    Crispy Chicken with Tomato
        Arugula Salad, 182–183
    Lemon-Basil Three Bean Salad,
        164
    Roasted Asparagus and Grape
        Tomatoes with Balsamic and
        Pecorino, 231
Banana Berry Ice Cream, 257
Banana Nutella Ice Cream, 257
Banana Nut Health Shake, 137
Banana Peanut Butter Ice Cream,
    257
bananas
    Baby Bump Banana Flax Bread, 73
    Banana Berry Ice Cream, 257
    Banana Nutella Ice Cream, 257
    Banana Nut Health Shake, 137
    Banana Peanut Butter Ice Cream,
        257
    Berrylicious Tofu Smoothie, 134
    Nutty for Chocolate Banana
        Smoothie, 136
    Nutty Nana No-Cook Overnight
        Oats, 95
    One-Ingredient Banana Ice
        Cream, 256–257
basil, Lemon-Basil Three Bean Salad,
    164
B-complex vitamins, micronutrients
    overview, 22. see also specific
    vitamins
beans. see specific types
beef
    Chipotle Burgers with Avocado
        Crema, 128–129

Grilled Skirt Steak with Chimichurri Sauce, 198
No More Takeout Beef with Broccoli, 196–197
Sunday Beef Stew, 200–201
Bellini, Baby, 140–141
berries. *see also specific types*
Banana Berry Ice Cream, 257
Berry and Ricotta Stuffed French Toast, 76
Berrylicious Tofu Smoothie, 134
Mixed Berry Crumble, 244
Sunshiny Day Breakfast Parfaits, 89
Berry and Ricotta Stuffed French Toast, 76
Berrylicious Tofu Smoothie, 134
beta-carotene, Vitamin A and, 22
beverages
Baby Bellini, 140–141
Banana Nut Health Shake, 137
Berrylicious Tofu Smoothie, 134
caffeine consumption, 19, 46–47
Cucumber Faux-jito, 142
Hydrating Honeydew Lemonade, 138–139
hydration and, 31, 53, 67
Mango Peach Blast, 138
Mariya's Green Smoothie, 136–137
morning sickness and, 32
Nutty for Chocolate Banana Smoothie, 136
Pineapple Ginger Spritzer, 141
Watermelon Agua Fresca, 139–140
birth defects
folate and, 17
Vitamin A and, 22
Black Bean and Quinoa Veggie Burgers, 126–128
black beans
Black Bean and Quinoa Veggie Burgers, 126–128
Easy Black Beans and Rice, 234
Lemon-Basil Three Bean Salad, 164
Pumpkin Turkey Chili, 187–188
Roasted Sweet Potato and Black Bean Tacos, 210–211
Blackberry Chia Jam, 87
Black Cod with Romesco Sauce, 181
blackstrap molasses, iron absorption and, 19
bleach solution for cleaning, 39
bloating and gas
fiber and, 12
tips for, 35–36
blood pressure, 29–30
blood sugar levels, 27–28, 50
blueberries
Baby on Board Blueberry Peach Cobbler, 242–243
Blueberry Maple Compote, 87
Blueberry Vanilla No-Cook Overnight Oats, 94
Buttermilk Blueberry Scookies, 254
Lemon Ricotta Blueberry Pancakes, 78–79

Rise and Shine Blueberry Oatmeal Muffins, 70–71
Blueberry Maple Compote, 87–88
Blueberry Vanilla No-Cook Overnight Oats, 94
BMI calculation, 6, 263–264
Bolognese, Spaghetti, 185–186
Brain-Boosting Salmon Burgers, 125–126
Braised Swiss Chard with White Beans, 221
BRAT diet, 32
bread-based recipes. *see also* appetizers, snacks, and sandwiches
Avocado Toast, 112
Berry and Ricotta Stuffed French Toast, 76
Chili Lime Avocado Toast, 112
Feta and Radish Avocado Toast, 113
Pan con Tomate (Tomato Bread), 106
Spinach, Mushroom, and Gruyere Breakfast Strata, 82–83
White Gazpacho, 151
breads
Baby Bump Banana Flax Bread, 73
Cauliflower Cheesy Bread, 104
essential foods, 59
breakfast
Almond Chia Pudding with Raspberries, 92
Almond Joy No-Cook Overnight Oats, 95
Apple Cinnamon Dutch Baby, 74
Baby Bump Banana Flax Bread, 73
Berry and Ricotta Stuffed French Toast, 76
Blackberry Chia Jam, 87–88
Blueberry Maple Compote, 87
Blueberry Vanilla No-Cook Overnight Oats, 94
Coconut Maple Granola, 86
healthy eating tips, 51–52
Lemon Ricotta Blueberry Pancakes, 78–79
Nutty Nana No-Cook Overnight Oats, 95
Peachy-Keen Baked Oatmeal, 84
"Pump Up Your Milk" Pumpkin Chocolate Chip Muffins, 72
Rise and Shine Blueberry Oatmeal Muffins, 70–71
Spinach, Mushroom, and Gruyere Breakfast Strata, 82–83
Strawberry Almond Breakfast Quinoa, 90
Summer Zucchini and Corn Frittata, 80–81
Sunshiny Day Breakfast Parfaits, 89
Turkey Sausage Egg White Flatbread, 79–80
breakfast cereals and folic acid, 52
breastfeeding
dietary reference intakes, 8, 265
protein requirements, 13, 28

brewer's yeast
"Pump Up Your Milk" Pumpkin Chocolate Chip Muffins, 72
broccoli
No More Takeout Beef with Broccoli, 196–197
Sesame Noodles with Broccoli, 108
Sesame Roasted Broccoli, 223
Brussels Sprouts, Miso Roasted, 220
burgers. *see* appetizers, snacks, and sandwiches
Butter Lettuce Salad with Buttermilk Herb Dressing, 156–157
buttermilk
Butter Lettuce Salad with Buttermilk Herb Dressing, 156–157
Buttermilk Blueberry Scookies, 254
Lemon Raspberry Buttermilk Popsicles, 258
Savory Tomato Cobbler, 236
Buttermilk Blueberry Scookies, 254
butternut squash
Roasted Butternut Squash Salad with Maple Dijon Vinaigrette, 160–161

C
cabbage
Caribbean Fish Tacos, 180
caffeine
foods to avoid or limit, 46–47
iron absorption and, 19
Cake, Fresh Strawberry, 248
calcium
iron absorption and, 19
micronutrients overview, 20
special diets and, 26
Vitamin D and, 21
cannellini beans
Braised Swiss Chard with White Beans, 221
Power-Packed Pasta Fagioli, 153–154
Cannoli Cream-Filled Strawberries, 243
canola oil, genetic engineering and, 56
capers
Pantry Pasta Puttanesca, 212
carbohydrates. *see also specific types*
fiber as, 12
healthy eating tips, 51
macronutrients overview, 8–11
simple vs. complex, 9
whole vs. refined grains, 9–11
Caribbean Fish Tacos, 180
Carrie's Experimental Kitchen, 79, 164
carrots
Comfort in a Bowl Carrot Ginger Soup, 148
cast-iron pans, for iron absorption, 19
Cauliflower Cheesy Bread, 104
Celery Root Puree, Autumn, 230
cereal grains. *see also specific types*
essential foods, 59–60

as fiber source, 12
folic acid and cereals, 52
chard
    Braised Swiss Chard with White
       Beans, 221
cheeses. *see also specific types*
    Cauliflower Cheesy Bread, 104
    Cheesy Quinoa and Bacon
       Casserole, 203
    essential foods, 62
    Green Grilled Cheese Sandwich,
       131
    pasteurization of, 44
    Spinach, Mushroom, and Gruyere
       Breakfast Strata, 82–83
Cheesy Quinoa and Bacon Casserole,
    203
cherries
    Cherry Lime Granita, 260
    No-Bake Chocolate Cherry Granola
       Bars, 110–111
Cherry Lime Granita, 260
chia seeds
    Almond Chia Pudding with
       Raspberries, 92
    Blackberry Chia Jam, 87
    "Pump Up Your Milk" Pumpkin
       Chocolate Chip Muffins, 72
chicken
    Balsamic, Maple, and Thyme
       Roasted Chicken, 194–195
    Chicken Salad with a Twist, 158
    Classic Chicken Noodle Soup, 146
    Creamy Paprika Chicken with Egg
       Noodles, 192
    Crispy Chicken with Tomato
       Arugula Salad, 182–183
    Greek Chicken Meatballs, 107
    Homemade Chicken Stock, 147
    Slow Cooker Pulled Chicken,
       183–184
Chicken Noodle Soup, Classic, 146
Chicken Salad with a Twist, 158
Chicken Stock, Homemade, 147
Chickpea and Spinach Curry, 208–209
chickpeas
    Chickpea and Spinach Curry, 208–
      209
    Crispy Spiced Chickpeas, 116
    Lemon-Basil Three Bean Salad, 164
    Simply Delicious Hummus, 114
Chili Lime Avocado Toast, 112
Chili, Pumpkin Turkey, 187–188
chill food safety step, 41–42
Chimichurri Sauce, Grilled Skirt Steak
    with, 198
Chipotle Burgers with Avocado Crema,
    128–129
chipotle peppers
    Chipotle Burgers with Avocado
       Crema, 128–129
    Pumpkin Turkey Chili, 187–188
    Roasted Sweet Potato Coins with
       Chipotle Crema, 98
chips

Crispy Kale Chips, 119
nutritional comparison, 4
chocolate
    Chunky Monkey Ice Cream, 257
    Craveable Chocolate Ganache
       Cupcakes, 250 251
    No-Bake Chocolate Cherry Granola
       Bars, 110–111
    Nutty for Chocolate Banana
       Smoothie, 136
    "Pump Up Your Milk" Pumpkin
       Chocolate Chip Muffins, 72
chocolate almond milk
    Almond Joy No-Cook Overnight
       Oats, 95
choline, micronutrients overview, 23
Chunky Monkey Ice Cream, 257
cider
    Baby Bellini, 140–141
    Cider Baked Apples, 246
    pasteurization of, 44
Cider Baked Apples, 246
Classic Chicken Noodle Soup, 146
clean food safety step, 38–39
club soda
    Cucumber Faux-jito, 142
    Pineapple Ginger Spritzer, 141
cobblers
    Baby on Board Blueberry Peach
       Cobbler, 242–243
    Savory Tomato Cobbler, 236
coconut and coconut milk
    Cider Baked Apples, 246
    Thai Red Curry Tofu, 214–215
Coconut Maple Granola, 86
cod
    Black Cod with Romesco Sauce, 181
coffee
    foods to avoid or limit, 46–47
    iron absorption and caffeine, 19
Comfort in a Bowl Carrot Ginger
    Soup, 148
Compote, Blueberry Maple, 87
constipation
    fiber and, 12
    tips for, 35–36
contamination
    avoiding, 39
    seafood, 43–44
cook food safety step, 40–41
cookies
    Buttermilk Blueberry Scookies, 254
    Flourless Peanut Butter Cookies,
      252
cooking tips. *see also* diet and nutrition
    background of book, vi–vii
    cook at home, vii, 55–57
    digestive issues, reducing, 35–36
    healthy techniques, 56
    plan your meals, 57–58
    stock your kitchen, 58–63
corn
    Butter Lettuce Salad with
       Buttermilk Herb Dressing,
       156–157

    Farro Salad with Corn, Tomatoes,
       and Edamame, 164–165
    Seared Scallops with Creamy Corn,
       174
    Summer Zucchini and Corn Frittata,
       80 81
corn tortillas
    Caribbean Fish Tacos, 180
    Roasted Sweet Potato and Black
       Bean Tacos, 210–211
Couscous Lentil Salad, 161–162
Craveable Chocolate Ganache
    Cupcakes, 250–251
cravings
    background of book, vi, 67
    controlling, 33–34
    healthy eating tips, 50
cream cheese
    Cannoli Cream-Filled Strawberries,
       243
    Creamy Paprika Chicken with Egg
       Noodles, 192
crema
    Chipotle Burgers with Avocado
       Crema, 128–129
    Cilantro Lime Crema, 210–211
    Roasted Sweet Potato Coins with
       Chipotle Crema, 98
Crispy Chicken with Tomato Arugula
    Salad, 182–183
Crispy Kale Chips, 119
Crispy Spiced Chickpeas, 116
cross-contamination, avoiding, 39
Crumble, Mixed Berry, 244
Cuban Mojo Pork Tenderloin, 204
Cucumber Faux-jito, 142
cucumbers
    Cucumber Faux-jito, 142
    Refrigerator Dill Pickles, 117
    White Gazpacho, 151
Cupcakes, Craveable Chocolate
    Ganache, 250–251
Curry, Chickpea and Spinach, 208 209
curry paste, Thai Red Curry Tofu,
    214 215
cutting boards, avoiding contamination,
    39

D
dairy products. *see also specific foods*
    essential foods, 62
    meal planning, 24–25
    pasteurization process, 44
    protein sources, 13
dehydration, avoiding, 31, 53
desserts
    Baby on Board Blueberry Peach
       Cobbler, 242–243
    Banana Berry Ice Cream, 257
    Banana Nutella Ice Cream, 257
    Banana Peanut Butter Ice Cream,
       257
    Buttermilk Blueberry Scookies, 254
    Cannoli Cream-Filled Strawberries,
       243

Cherry Lime Granita, 260
Chunky Monkey Ice Cream, 257
Cider Baked Apples, 246
Craveable Chocolate Ganache
     Cupcakes, 250–251
Flourless Peanut Butter Cookies,
     252
Fresh Strawberry Cake, 248
Honey Lemon Cookies, 252–253
Lemon Raspberry Buttermilk
     Popsicles, 258
Mixed Berry Crumble, 244
One-Ingredient Banana Ice Cream,
     256–257
Pumpkin Custard, 262
Rock-a-Bye Baby Roasted Apricots,
     247
Super-Fast Peach Frozen Yogurt,
     255
Deviled Egg Spread, 118
DHA (docosahexaeonic acid), 15–16
diabetes, 27–28
diet and nutrition
     background of book, v–vii
     BMI calculation, 6, 263–264
     breakfast cereals, 52
     cooking tips, 55–63
     dietary guidelines for seafood, 43
     dietary reference intakes, 8, 265
     eating for two, 3–23
     eating small, frequent meals, 50–52
     eating twice as smart, not twice as
          much, 4–5, 49–50
     eating well, 49–54
     essential foods, 58, 59–63
     food safety and what to avoid, 37–48
     healthy snack and meal ideas, 5,
          33–34, 51
     hydrating, 53
     introduction, 3–5
     macronutrients overview, 8–16
     meal planning, 24–28, 57–58
     micronutrients overview, 17–23
     side effects and, 29–36
     special diets overview, 26–28
     staying active, 54
     super foods, 50
     weight gain guidelines, 5–7
dietary reference intakes, 8, 265
dill
     Dill Yogurt Sauce, 125–126
     Refrigerator Dill Pickles, 117
Dill Yogurt Sauce, 125–126
docosahexaeonic acid (DHA), 15–16
Doxylamine, 31
dressings. see soups, salads, and
     dressings
dried fruit
     No-Bake Chocolate Cherry Granola
          Bars, 110–111
     Tropical Popcorn Trail Mix, 120
dried tomatoes
     Mediterranean Quinoa, 235
     Mediterranean Shrimp Pasta, 176
drinks. see beverages

Dutch Baby, Apple Cinnamon, 74

E
Easy Black Beans and Rice, 234
eating well. see diet and nutrition
edamame
     Farro Salad with Corn, Tomatoes,
          and Edamame, 164–165
     Wok-Charred Edamame with Sweet
          Soy Glaze, 100
eggplant
     Roasted Eggplant and Tomato Soup
          with Fresh Herbs, 152
eggs
     Deviled Egg Spread, 118
     essential foods, 62
     food safety, 39–41, 44
     Pumpkin Custard, 262
     Quinoa Fried "Rice," 232
     raw or undercooked, 44
     Spinach, Mushroom, and Gruyere
          Breakfast Strata, 82–83
     Summer Zucchini and Corn Frittata,
          80–81
     Turkey Sausage Egg White
          Flatbread, 79–80
eicosapentaenoic acid (EPA), 15–16
electrolytes overview, 22–23
emotional support, 34
enriched grains, defined, 11
entrées
     Balsamic, Maple, and Thyme
          Roasted Chicken, 194–195
     Black Cod with Romesco Sauce, 181
     Caribbean Fish Tacos, 180
     Cheesy Quinoa and Bacon
          Casserole, 203
     Chickpea and Spinach Curry, 208–
          209
     Creamy Paprika Chicken with Egg
          Noodles, 192
     Crispy Chicken with Tomato
          Arugula Salad, 182–183
     Cuban Mojo Pork Tenderloin, 204
     Grilled Skirt Steak with
          Chimichurri Sauce, 198
     Lemon Risotto with Spring
          Vegetables, 216–217
     Mediterranean Shrimp Pasta, 176
     No More Takeout Beef with
          Broccoli, 196–197
     Orecchiette with Kale and Turkey
          Sausage, 188–189
     Pantry Pasta Puttanesca, 212
     Pumpkin Turkey Chili, 187–188
     Quick and Easy Miso-Glazed
          Salmon, 168
     Roasted Sweet Potato and Black
          Bean Tacos, 210–211
     Rosemary and Lemon Grilled Lamb
          Chops, 202
     Salmon Oreganata, 178
     Seared Scallops with Creamy Corn,
          174
     Shrimp and Grits, 172–173

Shrimp and Sausage Jambalaya,
     171–172
Slow Cooker Pulled Chicken,
     183–184
Southwest Shepherd's Pie, 190–191
Spaghetti Bolognese, 185–186
Spaghetti Squash Lasagna, 206–207
Sunday Beef Stew, 200–201
Thai Red Curry Tofu, 214–215
Tilapia Piccata, 170
EPA (eicosapentaenoic acid), 15–16
equipment, kitchen, 58, 59
exercise
     benefits, 54
     constipation, bloating, and gas, 35
     cravings and, 33
     diabetes and, 28

F
family meal traditions, 56–57
Farro Salad with Corn, Tomatoes, and
     Edamame, 164–165
fats
     in Greek vs. regular yogurt, 14
     macronutrients overview, 14–16
     meal planning, 24–25
Faux-jito, Cucumber, 142
Feta and Radish Avocado Toast, 113
feta cheese
     Farro Salad with Corn, Tomatoes,
          and Edamame, 164–165
     Feta and Radish Avocado Toast, 113
     Greek Chicken Meatballs, 107
     Roasted Eggplant and Tomato Soup
          with Fresh Herbs, 152
     Roasted Sweet Potato and Black
          Bean Tacos, 180
fetal alcohol spectrum disorders, 48
fiber
     constipation, bloating, and gas, 35
     macronutrients overview, 12
FIFO (first in, first out) rule, 58
first trimester
     blood pressure, 29
     changes overview, vi, 30
     dietary reference intakes, 8
     folate requirements, 17
     meal plan example, 25
     weight gain, 6
fish. see also specific types
     Caribbean Fish Tacos, 180
     essential foods, 62
     food safety, 39–44
     as omega-3 source, 16
Flatbread, Turkey Sausage Egg White,
     79–80
flaxseed
     Baby Bump Banana Flax Bread, 73
     Banana Nut Health Shake, 137
     Flourless Peanut Butter Cookies,
          252
     Mango Peach Blast, 138
     No-Bake Chocolate Cherry Granola
          Bars, 110–111

"Pump Up Your Milk" Pumpkin
Chocolate Chip Muffins, 72
Flourless Peanut Butter Cookies, 252
fluid intake
constipation, bloating, and gas, 35
healthy eating tips, 53
morning sickness and, 32
folate
healthy eating tips, 52
micronutrients overview, 17–18
Food Done Light, 161, 252
food labels
fats, 15
pasteurization, 44
"sell by" dates, 41–42
"use by" dates, 58
whole grains, 11
food plans. see diet and nutrition; meal
planning
food preparation
cooking at home, 55–57
food safety, 38–42
food safety
chill step, 41–42
clean step, 38–39
cook step, 40–41
introduction, 37–38
meal planning, 58
separate step, 39
foods to avoid or limit
alcohol, 48
caffeine, 46–47
high mercury seafood, 42–43
raw or undercooked meat, poultry,
and eggs, 44
raw, undercooked, or contaminated
seafood, 43–44
unpasteurized foods, 44
unwashed fruits and vegetables,
45–46
food thermometers, 40–41
fortified grains, defined, 11
Fountain Avenue Kitchen, 118
France
alcohol warning labels, 48
pregnancy diet, 42
freezer
background of book, 67
essential foods, 63
meal planning, 58
postpartum diet, 28
French Toast, Berry and Ricotta
Stuffed, 76
Fresh Strawberry Cake, 248
Frittata, Summer Zucchini and Corn,
80–81
frozen desserts. see desserts
fruits. see also specific types
essential foods, 61, 63
as fiber source, 12
food safety, 39, 45–46
meal planning, 24–25
organic, 45–46
water content, 53
Full Belly Sisters, 72, 131

G
Gambas al Ajillo (Spanish Garlic
Shrimp), 102
Ganache, Chocolate, 250–251
garam masala
Chickpea and Spinach Curry, 208–
209
garlic
Pan con Tomate (Tomato Bread),
106
Quinoa Fried "Rice," 232
Sautéed Kale with Lemon and
Garlic, 222
Spanish Garlic Shrimp (Gambas al
Ajillo), 102
gas and bloating
fiber and, 12
tips for, 35–36
Gazpacho, White, 151
genetically modified organisms, 56
GERD (gastroesophageal reflux
disease), 36
gestational diabetes, 27–28
ginger
Comfort in a Bowl Carrot Ginger
Soup, 148
for morning sickness, 31
Pineapple Ginger Spritzer, 141
Quinoa Fried "Rice," 232
goat cheese. see also feta cheese
Quinoa Salad with Spinach,
Strawberries, and Goat Cheese,
159–160
Roasted Butternut Squash Salad
with Maple Dijon Vinaigrette,
160–161
Roasted Eggplant and Tomato Soup
with Fresh Herbs, 152
grains. see also specific types
essential foods, 59–60
as fiber source, 12
folic acid and cereals, 52
meal planning, 24–25
nutrition overview, 9–11
Granita, Cherry Lime, 260
Granola Bars, No-Bake Chocolate
Cherry, 110–111
Granola, Coconut Maple, 86
grapes
White Gazpacho, 151
Greek Chicken Meatballs, 107
Greek yogurt. see yogurt, Greek
Green Grilled Cheese Sandwich, 131
Green Smoothie, Mariya's, 136–137
Gremolata, Sage and Parmesan,
with Hasselback Sweet Potatoes,
228–229
Grilled Cheese Sandwich, Green, 131
Grilled Skirt Steak with Chimichurri
Sauce, 198
Grits, Shrimp and, 172–173
grocery lists, 58
Gruyere cheese, Spinach, Mushroom,
and Gruyere Breakfast Strata,
82–83

H
halibut
Caribbean Fish Tacos, 180
Hasselback Sweet Potatoes with Sage
and Parmesan Gremolata, 228–229
healthy eating. see diet and nutrition
heartburn, tips for, 36
heating of food, 41–42
heme iron form, 18–19
hemoglobin, iron and, 18
hemorrhoids, 12, 35
herbs, essential, 61
high mercury seafood, 42–43
Homemade Chicken Stock, 147
Homemade Vegan Mayonnaise,
123–124
honeydew melon
Hydrating Honeydew Lemonade,
138–139
Honey Lemon Cookies, 252–253
hummus
Roasted Vegetable Hummus Wraps,
124
Simply Delicious Hummus, 114
Hydrating Honeydew Lemonade,
138–139
hydration (of body), 31, 53, 67
hydrogenation process, 15
hygeine, food. see food safety
Hyperemesis gravidarum, 30

I
ice cream
Banana Berry Ice Cream, 257
Banana Nutella Ice Cream, 257
Banana Peanut Butter Ice Cream,
257
Chunky Monkey Ice Cream, 257
One-Ingredient Banana Ice Cream,
256–257
insulin, 27, 50
iodine, micronutrients overview, 23
iron
absorption tips, 19, 22
constipation, bloating, and gas, 35
micronutrients overview, 18–19
morning sickness, 31
Italian Lentil Soup, 150

J
Jambalaya, Shrimp and Sausage,
171–172
Jam, Blackberry Chia, 87
Japan, pregnancy diet, 42
jicama
Tropical Shrimp Salad, 162–163

K
kale
Crispy Kale Chips, 119
Mariya's Green Smoothie, 136–137
Orecchiette with Kale and Turkey
Sausage, 188–189

Power-Packed Pasta Fagioli, 153–154

Sautéed Kale with Lemon and Garlic, 222

Tuscan Kale and Apple Salad, 154–155

kidney beans

Braised Swiss Chard with White Beans, 221

Lemon-Basil Three Bean Salad, 164

Power-Packed Pasta Fagioli, 153–154

kitchen supplies

background of book, vii

essential foods, 58, 59–63

essential tools, 58, 59

L

lacto-ovo vegetarian diets, 27. *see also* vegetarian diets

lactose intolerance, 20, 27

lacto-vegetarian diets, 27. *see also* vegetarian diets

lamb

Rosemary and Lemon Grilled Lamb Chops, 202

Lasagna, Spaghetti Squash, 206–207

Lauren Kelly Nutrition, 203, 252

lean proteins, choosing, 13

legumes. *see also specific types*

essential foods, 60

as fiber source, 12

Lemonade, Hydrating Honeydew, 138–139

Lemon-Basil Three Bean Salad, 164

Lemon Raspberry Buttermilk Popsicles, 258

Lemon Ricotta Blueberry Pancakes, 78–79

Lemon Risotto with Spring Vegetables, 216–217

lemons and lemon juice

Honey Lemon Cookies, 252–253

Hydrating Honeydew Lemonade, 138–139

Lemon-Basil Three Bean Salad, 164

Lemon Raspberry Buttermilk Popsicles, 258

Lemon Ricotta Blueberry Pancakes, 78–79

Lemon Risotto with Spring Vegetables, 216–217

Rosemary and Lemon Grilled Lamb Chops, 202

Sautéed Kale with Lemon and Garlic, 222

lentils

Couscous Lentil Salad, 161–162

Italian Lentil Soup, 150

lettuce

Butter Lettuce Salad with Buttermilk Herb Dressing, 156–157

Tropical Shrimp Salad, 162–163

limes and lime juice

Cherry Lime Granita, 260

Chili Lime Avocado Toast, 112

Cilantro Lime Crema, 210–211

Cuban Mojo Pork Tenderloin, 204

Cucumber Faux-jito, 142

Listeria monocytogenes, 38

liver toxicity, Vitamin A and, 22

M

macronutrients overview. *see also specific types*

carbohydrates, 8–11

fats, 14–16

fiber, 12

macronutrients defined, 8

protein, 13–14

whole vs. refined grains, 9–11

main dishes. *see* entrées

Mango Peach Blast, 138

mangos

Mango Peach Blast, 138

Mariya's Green Smoothie, 136–137

Tropical Shrimp Salad, 162–163

Maple Dijon Vinaigrette, Roasted Butternut Squash Salad with, 160–161

Maple-Glazed Acorn Squash, 227

Maple Mashed Sweet Potatoes, 229

maple syrup

Balsamic, Maple, and Thyme Roasted Chicken, 194–195

Blueberry Maple Compote, 87

Coconut Maple Granola, 86

Maple-Glazed Acorn Squash, 227

Maple Mashed Sweet Potatoes, 229

Roasted Butternut Squash Salad with Maple Dijon Vinaigrette, 160–161

marinara sauce

Turkey Parmesan Burgers, 130

Mariya's Green Smoothie, 136–137

Mayonnaise, Homemade Vegan, 123–124

meal planning. *see also* diet and nutrition

background of book, vi–vii

gestational diabetes, 27–28

healthy cooking tips, 57–58

lactose intolerance, 27

MyPlate, 24–25

postpartum diet, 28

vegetarian diets, 26–27

meat. *see also specific types*

essential foods, 62

food safety, 39–41, 44

iron sources, 19

protein sources, 13

Meatballs, Greek Chicken, 107

Mediterranean Quinoa, 235

Mediterranean Shrimp Pasta, 176

melons

Hydrating Honeydew Lemonade, 138–139

Mariya's Green Smoothie, 136–137

Watermelon Agua Fresca, 139–140

mercury in seafood, 42–43

micronutrients overview. *see also specific types*

B-complex vitamins, 22

calcium, 20

choline, 23

folate, 17–18

iodine, 23

iron, 18–19

micronutrients defined, 8

sodium and potassium, 22–23

Vitamin A, 22

Vitamin C, 22

Vitamin D, 21

zinc, 23

milk, almond

Almond Chia Pudding with Raspberries, 92

Almond Joy No-Cook Overnight Oats, 95

Banana Nut Health Shake, 137

Blueberry Vanilla No-Cook Overnight Oats, 94

Nutty Nana No-Cook Overnight Oats, 95

Peachy-Keen Baked Oatmeal, 84

Strawberry Almond Breakfast Quinoa, 90

milk, dairy

Autumn Celery Root Puree, 230

Banana Berry Ice Cream, 257

Blueberry Vanilla No-Cook Overnight Oats, 94

Cheesy Quinoa and Bacon Casserole, 203

essential foods, 62

Nutty for Chocolate Banana Smoothie, 136

Nutty Nana No-Cook Overnight Oats, 95

pasteurization of, 44

Peachy-Keen Baked Oatmeal, 84

Pumpkin Custard, 262

Roasted Eggplant and Tomato Soup with Fresh Herbs, 152

Spaghetti Bolognese, 185–186

minerals overview. *see* micronutrients overview

mint

Cucumber Faux-jito, 142

miso paste

Miso Roasted Brussels Sprouts, 220

Quick and Easy Miso-Glazed Salmon, 168

Miso Roasted Brussels Sprouts, 220

Mixed Berry Crumble, 244

molasses, iron absorption and, 19

monounsaturated fats, 14–15

morning sickness

background of book, vi, vii, 67

prevalence and symptoms, 30

tips for, 31–32

mozzarella cheese

Spaghetti Squash Lasagna, 206–207

muffins

"Pump Up Your Milk" Pumpkin Chocolate Chip Muffins, 72
Rise and Shine Blueberry Oatmeal Muffins, 70–71
mushrooms
Creamy Paprika Chicken with Egg Noodles, 192
Spinach, Mushroom, and Gruyere Breakfast Strata, 82–83
Sunday Beef Stew, 200–201
MyPlate, 24–25

N
nausea and vomiting. *see* morning sickness
neural tube defects, folate and, 17
No-Bake Chocolate Cherry Granola Bars, 110–111
No More Takeout Beef with Broccoli, 196–197
non-heme iron form, 18
noodles. *see also* pasta
Classic Chicken Noodle Soup, 146
Creamy Paprika Chicken with Egg Noodles, 192
Sesame Noodles with Broccoli, 108
Nutella, Banana Nutella Ice Cream, 257
nutrition. *see* diet and nutrition
nutrition labels. *see* food labels
nuts. *see also specific types*
essential foods, 60
as fiber source, 12
Snack Attack Spiced Nuts, 122
Tropical Popcorn Trail Mix, 120
Nutty for Chocolate Banana Smoothie, 136
Nutty Nana No-Cook Overnight Oats, 95

O
oats and oatmeal
Almond Joy No-Cook Overnight Oats, 95
Banana Nut Health Shake, 137
Black Bean and Quinoa Veggie Burgers, 126–128
Blueberry Vanilla No-Cook Overnight Oats, 94
Cider Baked Apples, 246
Flourless Peanut Butter Cookies, 252
Mixed Berry Crumble, 244
No-Bake Chocolate Cherry Granola Bars, 110–111
Nutty Nana No-Cook Overnight Oats, 95
Peachy-Keen Baked Oatmeal, 84
Rise and Shine Blueberry Oatmeal Muffins, 70–71
oils
essential foods, 60
for healthy cooking, 56
meal planning, 24–25

olive oil for healthy cooking, 56
olives
Pantry Pasta Puttanesca, 212
omega-3 fatty acids, 15–16, 42
One-Ingredient Banana Ice Cream, 256–257
orange juice
Berrylicious Tofu Smoothie, 134
Comfort in a Bowl Carrot Ginger Soup, 148
Cuban Mojo Pork Tenderloin, 204
Mango Peach Blast, 138
Orecchiette with Kale and Turkey Sausage, 188–189
Oreganata, Salmon, 178
organic foods, 62
organic produce, 45–46
Oven-Roasted Vegetables, 224
ovo vegetarian diets, 27. *see also* vegetarian diets

P
pancakes
Apple Cinnamon Dutch Baby, 74
Lemon Ricotta Blueberry Pancakes, 78–79
Pan con Tomate (Tomato Bread), 106
pans, cast iron, 19
pantry, essential foods, 59–61
Pantry Pasta Puttanesca, 212
Paprika Chicken, Creamy, with Egg Noodles, 192
Parfaits, Sunshiny Day Breakfast, 89
Parmesan cheese
Preggo Parmesan and Herb Popovers, 238
Turkey Parmesan Burgers, 130
Parmigiano-Reggiano cheese
Hasselback Sweet Potatoes with Sage and Parmesan Gremolata, 228–229
Lemon Risotto with Spring Vegetables, 216–217
Mediterranean Shrimp Pasta, 176
Orecchiette with Kale and Turkey Sausage, 188–189
Roasted Asparagus and Grape Tomatoes with Balsamic and Pecorino, 231
Spaghetti Squash Lasagna, 206–207
Summer Zucchini and Corn Frittata, 80–81
Tuscan Kale and Apple Salad, 154–155
partially hydrogenated fats, 15
pasta. *see also* noodles
as fiber source, 12
Mediterranean Shrimp Pasta, 176
Orecchiette with Kale and Turkey Sausage, 188–189
Pantry Pasta Puttanesca, 212
Power-Packed Pasta Fagioli, 153–154
Sesame Noodles with Broccoli, 108
Spaghetti Bolognese, 185–186

Pasta Fagioli, Power-Packed, 153–154
pasteurization process, 44
pathogens in food. *see* food safety
peaches
Baby Bellini, 140–141
Baby on Board Blueberry Peach Cobbler, 242–243
Mango Peach Blast, 138
Peachy-Keen Baked Oatmeal, 84
Super-Fast Peach Frozen Yogurt, 255
Peachy-Keen Baked Oatmeal, 84
peanut butter
Banana Peanut Butter Ice Cream, 257
Flourless Peanut Butter Cookies, 252
Nutty for Chocolate Banana Smoothie, 136
Nutty Nana No-Cook Overnight Oats, 95
Sesame Noodles with Broccoli, 108
pecans
Baby Bump Banana Flax Bread, 73
Cider Baked Apples, 246
Mixed Berry Crumble, 244
Roasted Butternut Squash Salad with Maple Dijon Vinaigrette, 160–161
Pecorino Romano cheese
Orecchiette with Kale and Turkey Sausage, 188–189
Roasted Asparagus and Grape Tomatoes with Balsamic and Pecorino, 231
pesticide residues, 45–46
physical activity. *see* exercise
pica, 33
Piccata, Tilapia, 170
Pickled Shallots, Quick, 123
Pickles, Refrigerator Dill, 117
Pineapple Ginger Spritzer, 141
plant sources of protein, 13
polyunsaturated fats, 14–16
popcorn
Tropical Popcorn Trail Mix, 120
Popovers, Preggo Parmesan and Herb, 238
Popsicles, Lemon Raspberry Buttermilk, 258
pork
Cheesy Quinoa and Bacon Casserole, 203
Cuban Mojo Pork Tenderloin, 204
postpartum diet, 28
potassium, micronutrients overview, 22–23
potato chips, nutritional information, 4
potatoes, sweet
Hasselback Sweet Potatoes with Sage and Parmesan Gremolata, 228–229
Maple Mashed Sweet Potatoes, 229
Roasted Sweet Potato and Black Bean Tacos, 210–211

Roasted Sweet Potato Coins with
  Chipotle Crema, 98
Southwest Shepherd's Pie, 190–191
Sweet Potato Fries, 226
potatoes, white
  Autumn Celery Root Puree, 230
poultry. see also specific types
  essential foods, 62
  food safety, 39–41, 44
Power-Packed Pasta Fagioli, 153–154
preeclampsia, symptoms, 20, 30
Preggo Parmesan and Herb Popovers,
  238
prenatal vitamins overview. see
  micronutrients overview
progesterone, 35–36
protein
  healthy eating tips, 50–51
  macronutrients overview, 13–14
  meal planning, 24–25
  morning sickness and, 32
  postpartum diet, 26
Pudding, Almond Chia, with
  Raspberries, 92
puffed rice cereal, No-Bake Chocolate
  Cherry Granola Bars, 110–111
pumpkin
  Pumpkin Custard, 262
  Pumpkin Turkey Chili, 187–188
  "Pump Up Your Milk" Pumpkin
    Chocolate Chip Muffins, 72
Pumpkin Custard, 262
Pumpkin Turkey Chili, 187–188
"Pump Up Your Milk" Pumpkin
  Chocolate Chip Muffins, 72
Puttanesca, Pantry Pasta, 212

Q
Quick and Easy Miso-Glazed Salmon,
  168
Quick Pickled Shallots, 123
quinoa
  Black Bean and Quinoa Veggie
    Burgers, 126–128
  Cheesy Quinoa and Bacon
    Casserole, 203
  Mediterranean Quinoa, 235
  Quinoa Fried "Rice," 232
  Quinoa Salad with Spinach,
    Strawberries, and Goat Cheese,
    159–160
  Strawberry Almond Breakfast
    Quinoa, 90
Quinoa Fried "Rice," 232
Quinoa Salad with Spinach,
  Strawberries, and Goat Cheese,
  159–160

R
radishes
  Feta and Radish Avocado Toast, 113
raspberries
  Almond Chia Pudding with
    Raspberries, 92

Baby Bellini, 140–141
Lemon Raspberry Buttermilk
  Popsicles, 258
raw or undercooked foods
  meat, poultry, and eggs, 44
  seafood, 43–44
refined grains, defined, 9, 11
reflux disease, 36
refrigerator
  essential foods, 62–63
  food safety, 39, 41–42
  meal planning, 58
Refrigerator Dill Pickles, 117
rest, cravings and, 34
rice cereal, No-Bake Chocolate Cherry
  Granola Bars, 110–111
Rice, Easy Black Beans, 234
ricotta
  Berry and Ricotta Stuffed French
    Toast, 76
  Cannoli Cream-Filled Strawberries,
    243
  Lemon Ricotta Blueberry Pancakes,
    78–79
  Spaghetti Squash Lasagna, 206–207
Rise and Shine Blueberry Oatmeal
  Muffins, 70–71
Risotto, Lemon, with Spring
  Vegetables, 216–217
Roasted Asparagus and Grape
  Tomatoes with Balsamic and
  Pecorino, 231
Roasted Butternut Squash Salad with
  Maple Dijon Vinaigrette, 160–161
Roasted Eggplant and Tomato Soup
  with Fresh Herbs, 152
Roasted Sweet Potato and Black Bean
  Tacos, 210–211
Roasted Sweet Potato Coins with
  Chipotle Crema, 98
Roasted Vegetable Hummus Wraps,
  124
Rock-a-Bye Baby Roasted Apricots,
  247
Romesco Sauce, Black Cod with, 181
Rosemary and Lemon Grilled Lamb
  Chops, 202

S
sablefish
  Black Cod with Romesco Sauce, 181
Sage and Parmesan Gremolata,
  Hasselback Sweet Potatoes with,
  228–229
salads. see soups, salads, and dressings
salmon
  Brain-Boosting Salmon Burgers,
    125–126
  Quick and Easy Miso-Glazed
    Salmon, 168
  Salmon Oreganata, 178
Salmon Oreganata, 178
salt, as iodine source, 23
sandwiches. see appetizers, snacks, and
  sandwiches

saturated fats, 14–15
sausage, turkey
  Orecchiette with Kale and Turkey
    Sausage, 188–189
  Shrimp and Sausage Jambalaya,
    171–172
  Turkey Sausage Egg White
    Flatbread, 79–80
Sautéed Kale with Lemon and Garlic,
  222
Savory Tomato Cobbler, 236
Scallops, Seared, with Creamy Corn,
  174
Scookies, Buttermilk Blueberry, 254
seafood. see also fish; specific types
  essential foods, 62
  food safety, 39–44
Seared Scallops with Creamy Corn,
  174
second trimester
  blood pressure, 29
  changes overview, vi
  cravings, 33
  dietary reference intakes, 8
  meal plan example, 25
  weight gain, 6
seeds. see also specific types
  essential foods, 60
  as fiber source, 12
"sell by" dates, 41–42
separate food safety step, 39
Sesame Noodles with Broccoli, 108
Sesame Roasted Broccoli, 223
sesame seeds
  Sesame Noodles with Broccoli, 108
  Sesame Roasted Broccoli, 223
shakes. see beverages
Shallots, Quick Pickled, 123
Shepherd's Pie, Southwest, 190–191
Sherry Vinaigrette, 165
shrimp
  Mediterranean Shrimp Pasta, 176
  Shrimp and Grits, 172–173
  Shrimp and Sausage Jambalaya,
    171–172
  Spanish Garlic Shrimp (Gambas al
    Ajillo), 102
  Tropical Shrimp Salad, 162–163
Shrimp and Grits, 172–173
Shrimp and Sausage Jambalaya,
  171–172
side dishes
  Autumn Celery Root Puree, 230
  Braised Swiss Chard with White
    Beans, 221
  Easy Black Beans and Rice, 234
  Hasselback Sweet Potatoes with
    Sage and Parmesan Gremolata,
    228–229
  Maple-Glazed Acorn Squash, 227
  Maple Mashed Sweet Potatoes, 229
  Mediterranean Quinoa, 235
  Miso Roasted Brussels Sprouts, 220
  Oven-Roasted Vegetables, 224

Preggo Parmesan and Herb
    Popovers, 238
Quinoa Fried "Rice," 232
Roasted Asparagus and Grape
    Tomatoes with Balsamic and
    Pecorino, 231
Sautéed Kale with Lemon and
    Garlic, 222
Savory Tomato Cobbler, 236
Sesame Roasted Broccoli, 223
Sweet Potato Fries, 226
side effects of pregnancy
    background of book, vi, vii, 67
    constipation, bloating, and gas,
        35–36
    cravings, 33–34
    fiber and, 12
    healthy eating tips, 50
    heartburn, 36
    introduction, 30–31
    morning sickness, 30–32
Simply Delicious Hummus, 114
Slow Cooker Pulled Chicken,
    183–184
smells
    food safety and, 42
    morning sickness and, 31
smoothies. see beverages
Snack Attack Spiced Nuts, 122
snacks. see appetizers, snacks, and
    sandwiches
sodium, micronutrients overview,
    22–23
soups, salads, and dressings
    Butter Lettuce Salad with
        Buttermilk Herb Dressing,
        156–157
    Buttermilk Herb Dressing, 156–157
    Chicken Salad with a Twist, 158
    Classic Chicken Noodle Soup, 146
    Comfort in a Bowl Carrot Ginger
        Soup, 148
    Couscous Lentil Salad, 161–162
    Farro Salad with Corn, Tomatoes,
        and Edamame, 164–165
    Homemade Chicken Stock, 147
    Italian Lentil Soup, 150
    Lemon-Basil Three Bean Salad, 164
    Power-Packed Pasta Fagioli, 153–
        154
    Quinoa Salad with Spinach,
        Strawberries, and Goat Cheese,
        159–160
    Roasted Butternut Squash Salad
        with Maple Dijon Vinaigrette,
        160–161
    Roasted Eggplant and Tomato Soup
        with Fresh Herbs, 152
    Tomato Arugula Salad, 182–183
    Tropical Shrimp Salad, 162–163
    Tuscan Kale and Apple Salad,
        154–155
    White Gazpacho, 151
sour cream

Roasted Sweet Potato Coins with
    Chipotle Crema, 98
Southwest Shepherd's Pie, 190–191
soy proteins, essential foods, 62
soy sauce
    Sesame Noodles with Broccoli, 108
    Wok-Charred Edamame with
        Sweet Soy Glaze, 100
spaghetti
    Mediterranean Shrimp Pasta, 176
    Sesame Noodles with Broccoli, 108
    Spaghetti Bolognese, 185–186
Spaghetti Bolognese, 185–186
Spaghetti Squash Lasagna, 206–207
Spanish Garlic Shrimp (Gambas al
    Ajillo), 102
Spiced Chickpeas, Crispy, 116
Spiced Nuts, Snack Attack, 122
spices, essential, 60
spinach
    Cheesy Quinoa and Bacon
        Casserole, 203
    Chickpea and Spinach Curry,
        208–209
    Greek Chicken Meatballs, 107
    Green Grilled Cheese Sandwich,
        131
    Mariya's Green Smoothie, 136–137
    Mediterranean Quinoa, 235
    Mediterranean Shrimp Pasta, 176
    Quinoa Salad with Spinach,
        Strawberries, and Goat Cheese,
        159–160
    Roasted Butternut Squash Salad
        with Maple Dijon Vinaigrette,
        160–161
    Roasted Vegetable Hummus Wraps,
        124
    Spaghetti Squash Lasagna, 206–207
    Spinach, Mushroom, and Gruyere
        Breakfast Strata, 82–83
Spinach, Mushroom, and Gruyere
    Breakfast Strata, 82–83
Spritzer, Pineapple Ginger, 141
squash
    Maple-Glazed Acorn Squash, 227
    Roasted Butternut Squash Salad
        with Maple Dijon Vinaigrette,
        160–161
    Spaghetti Squash Lasagna, 206–207
Stew, Sunday Beef, 200–201
Strata, Spinach, Mushroom, and
    Gruyere Breakfast, 82–83
strawberries
    Banana Berry Ice Cream, 257
    Cannoli Cream-Filled Strawberries,
        243
    Fresh Strawberry Cake, 248
    Mariya's Green Smoothie, 136–137
    Quinoa Salad with Spinach,
        Strawberries, and Goat Cheese,
        159–160
    Strawberry Almond Breakfast
        Quinoa, 90

Strawberry Almond Breakfast Quinoa,
    90
sugars
    blood sugar levels, 27–28, 50
    healthy eating tips, 51
    macronutrients overview, 9
Summer Zucchini and Corn Frittata,
    80–81
Sumptuous Spoonfuls, 152
Sunday Beef Stew, 200–201
sun-dried tomatoes
    Mediterranean Quinoa, 235
    Mediterranean Shrimp Pasta, 176
sun exposure, Vitamin D and, 21
Sunshiny Day Breakfast Parfaits, 89
Super-Fast Peach Frozen Yogurt, 255
sweeteners, essential, 60
sweet potatoes
    Hasselback Sweet Potatoes with
        Sage and Parmesan Gremolata,
        228–229
    Maple Mashed Sweet Potatoes, 229
    Roasted Sweet Potato and Black
        Bean Tacos, 210–211
    Roasted Sweet Potato Coins with
        Chipotle Crema, 98
    Southwest Shepherd's Pie, 190–191
    Sweet Potato Fries, 226
Sweet Potato Fries, 226
Swiss Chard, Braised, with White
    Beans, 221

T
tacos
    Caribbean Fish Tacos, 180
    Roasted Sweet Potato and Black
        Bean Tacos, 210–211
tahini paste
    Couscous Lentil Salad, 161–162
    Simply Delicious Hummus, 114
tea
    foods to avoid or limit, 46–47
    iron absorption and caffeine, 19
temperature of food, 40–44
Thai Red Curry Tofu, 214–215
thawing guidelines, 41
thermometers, 40–41
third trimester
    blood pressure, 29
    calcium requirements, 20
    changes overview, vi, 30
    constipation, bloating, and gas, 35
    DHA and, 15
    dietary reference intakes, 8
    heartburn, 36
    meal plan example, 25
    weight gain, 6
thyme, Balsamic, Maple, and Thyme
    Roasted Chicken, 194–195
Tilapia Piccata, 170
toast
    Avocado Toast, 112
    Chili Lime Avocado Toast, 112
    Feta and Radish Avocado Toast,
        113

tofu
Berrylicious Tofu Smoothie, 134
Homemade Vegan Mayonnaise, 123–124
Thai Red Curry Tofu, 214–215
Tomato Bread (Pan con Tomate), 106
tomatoes
Butter Lettuce Salad with Buttermilk Herb Dressing, 156–157
Crispy Chicken with Tomato Arugula Salad, 182–183
Farro Salad with Corn, Tomatoes, and Edamame, 164–165
Mediterranean Quinoa, 235
Mediterranean Shrimp Pasta, 176
Pan con Tomate (Tomato Bread), 106
Roasted Asparagus and Grape Tomatoes with Balsamic and Pecorino, 231
Roasted Eggplant and Tomato Soup with Fresh Herbs, 152
Savory Tomato Cobbler, 236
tools, kitchen, 58, 59
tortillas, corn
Cilantro Lime Crema, 210–211
Roasted Sweet Potato and Black Bean Tacos, 180
Trail Mix, Tropical Popcorn, 120
trans fats, 14–15
Tropical Popcorn Trail Mix, 120
Tropical Shrimp Salad, 162–163
turkey, ground
Pumpkin Turkey Chili, 187–188
Southwest Shepherd's Pie, 190–191
Spaghetti Bolognese, 185–186
Turkey Parmesan Burgers, 130
Turkey Parmesan Burgers, 130
turkey sausage
Orecchiette with Kale and Turkey Sausage, 188–189
Shrimp and Sausage Jambalaya, 171–172
Turkey Sausage Egg White Flatbread, 79–80
Turkey Sausage Egg White Flatbread, 79–80
Tuscan Kale and Apple Salad, 154–155

U
undercooked or raw foods
meat, poultry, and eggs, 44
seafood, 43–44
United States, pregnancy diet, 42
unpasteurized foods, 44
unsaturated fats, 14–15
unwashed produce, food safety, 45–46
"use by" dates, 58

V
vegan diets, 27. see also vegetarian diets
Vegan Mayonnaise, Homemade, 123–124

vegetables. see also specific types
calcium sources, 20
essential foods, 61, 63
as fiber source, 12
food safety, 39, 45–46
Lemon Risotto with Spring Vegetables, 216–217
meal planning, 24–25
organic, 45–46
Oven-Roasted Vegetables, 224
Roasted Vegetable Hummus Wraps, 124
water content, 53
vegetarian diets
iron sources, 19
meal planning, 26–27
omega-3 sources, 16
protein sources, 13, 26
types of, 27
Veggie Burgers, Black Bean and Quinoa, 126–128
vinaigrettes. see soups, salads, and dressings
vinegars, essential foods, 60. see also balsamic vinegar
Vitamin A, micronutrients overview, 22
Vitamin B complex, 23
Vitamin B$_6$, for morning sickness, 31
Vitamin B$_{12}$, meal planning, 26
Vitamin C
iron absorption and, 19, 22
micronutrients overview, 22
Vitamin D, micronutrients overview, 21
vitamins overview. see micronutrients overview
vomiting and nausea. see morning sickness

W
walnuts
Baby Bump Banana Flax Bread, 73
Chunky Monkey Ice Cream, 257
Cider Baked Apples, 246
washing, as food safety step, 38–39, 45–46
water consumption
constipation, bloating, and gas, 35
hydration and, 53
watermelon
Mariya's Green Smoothie, 136–137
Watermelon Agua Fresca, 139–140
Watermelon Agua Fresca, 139–140
water, sparkling
Cucumber Faux-jito, 142
Pineapple Ginger Spritzer, 141
weight gain
background of book, vi
BMI calculation, 6, 263–264
distribution of weight, 7
guidelines, 5–7
healthy eating tips, 49–50
wheat germ
No-Bake Chocolate Cherry Granola Bars, 110–111

Rise and Shine Blueberry Oatmeal Muffins, 70–71
White Gazpacho, 151
whole grains. see also specific types
defined, 9, 11
reading labels, 11
tips to increase, 10
Whole Grain Stamp, 11
Wok-Charred Edamame with Sweet Soy Glaze, 100
Wraps, Roasted Vegetable Hummus, 124
wrist bands, acupressure, 31

Y
yogurt, Greek
Almond Chia Pudding with Raspberries, 92
Baby Bump Banana Flax Bread, 73
Blueberry Vanilla No-Cook Overnight Oats, 94
Butter Lettuce Salad with Buttermilk Herb Dressing, 156–157
Chipotle Burgers with Avocado Crema, 128–129
Cilantro Lime Crema, 210–211
Dill Yogurt Sauce, 125–126
essential foods, 62
Fresh Strawberry Cake, 248
Honey Lemon Cookies, 252–253
Mango Peach Blast, 138
Mariya's Green Smoothie, 136–137
as protein source, 14
Rise and Shine Blueberry Oatmeal Muffins, 70–71
Roasted Sweet Potato Coins with Chipotle Crema, 98
Summer Zucchini and Corn Frittata, 80–81
Sunshiny Day Breakfast Parfaits, 89
Super-Fast Peach Frozen Yogurt, 255
Yogurt Sauce, 127
Yogurt Sauce, 127

Z
za'atar
Chicken Salad with a Twist, 158
Simply Delicious Hummus, 114
zinc, micronutrients overview, 23
zucchini
Summer Zucchini and Corn Frittata, 80–81